# Sexuality and Dementia

Also by Douglas Wornell, MD

*Wandering Explorers: Practical Dementia for Families and Caregivers*

# Sexuality and Dementia

## Compassionate and Practical Strategies for Dealing with Unexpected or Inappropriate Behaviors

DOUGLAS WORNELL, MD

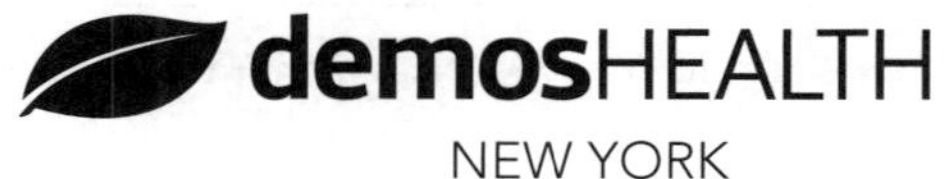


NEW YORK

**Visit our website at www.demoshealth.com**

*ISBN:* 978-1-936303-55-7
*e-book ISBN:* 978-1-61705-190-6

*Acquisitions Editor:* Julia Pastore
*Compositor:* diacriTech



**Library of Congress Cataloging-in-Publication Data**

Wornell, Douglas.
Sexuality and dementia : compassionate and practical strategies for dealing with unexpected or inappropriate behaviors / Douglas Wornell, MD.
pages cm
Includes bibliographical references and index.
ISBN 978-1-936303-55-7 (alk. paper)
1. Dementia—Patients—Sexual behavior. I. Title.
RC521.W67 2014
616.8′3—dc23

2013034850



Special Sales Department
Demos Medical Publishing, LLC
11 West 42nd Street, 15th Floor
New York, NY 10036
Phone: 800-532-8663 or 212-683-0072
Fax: 212-941-7842
E-mail: specialsales@demosmedpub.com

Printed in the United States of America by McNaughton & Gunn
13 14 15 16 17 / 5 4 3 2 1

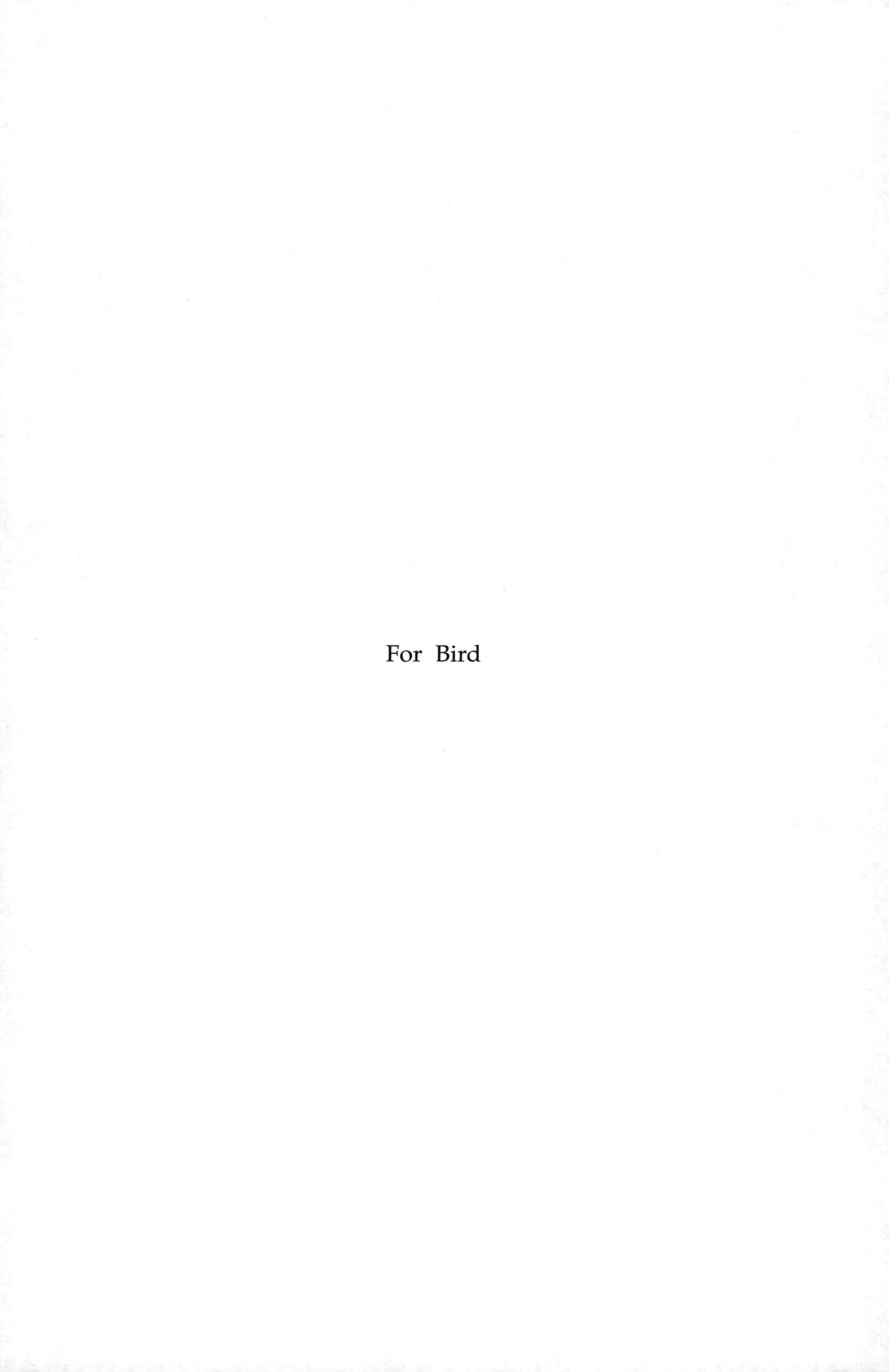

For Bird

# Contents

# Preface

## IS IT SEX—OR SOMETHING ELSE?

A recurring topic in my conversations with families and caregivers is whether or not we are actually talking about sexual activity when people with dementia reach out to one another, or to others. Sex is by definition a mix of emotion and physiology. That is, sexual thoughts and interest are followed by bodily arousal and ultimately sexual activity. Yet we are not neurobiological experiments walking around. Our sexual psychology and physical reactions vary and are often cloaked by several other factors such as culture, the current social situation, and life experience. At times this uncertainty of what another might be feeling sexually adds to the excitement. At other times it results in fear. It is at the core of receiving flirtation, for example, to try and decipher whether or not someone is interested and hinting sexually or just making some other, less intimate, contact. And then there are other situations, such as in the case of perversion or stalking, where the excitement is replaced by a very negative "creepy" feeling.

So what about our reaction to those with dementia, hidden sexually in a world of confusion? We know that dementia in general diminishes sexual behavior. There's just less brain, less testosterone, less everything to get things going. Yet we also know that social inhibitions falter, that psychosis and paranoia create chaos in relationships, that certain medications or lesions may actually lead to an increase in sexual activity in dementia patients, and that partners are left devastated and trying to deal with their own emotions. Still, that's not the whole story. There is something missing here, something big and unclear. What about the people with advancing neurological disease who are transitioning downwards, memory by memory, ability by ability, who still have some need to touch, to hug, to kiss? Yes, some may be openly flirtatious and others perverse, but the majority just seem to be what we might imagine ourselves to be if in their shoes. Are they feeling sexual? Or are they lonely, locked away in a disease, living in their past and far away from their present? Just wanting to connect...somehow, with someone? That is the something else. The something big.

Behavior can be interpreted in as many different ways as there are individuals observing it. What a spouse interprets as tenderness, a caregiver may view as overtly sexual. What one facility determines is acceptable touch, another may censure. What might be labeled as "just the need to touch" by a doctor might still be very sexual to the long-time romantic partner. What follows are many stories of patients and caregivers and spouses—each with their own needs and interpretations. Hopefully, these will be of benefit to others navigating this experience.

PART ONE

# A Different View of Sexual Behavior

CHAPTER ONE

# An Unexpected Symptom: A Very Common Occurrence

The first time I met with Kate and John, a silver-haired and healthy-looking couple in their early 70s, I was not surprised by the story Kate told me. John, big and bearish but gentle, who had been diagnosed with dementia several months before, was a retired OB-GYN. Kate, a petite live wire, was clearly worried about him. Exhausted, she sat by her husband's side. Both of them look dazed and confused, angry and frightened. It only took a glance into their eyes to see that this was not where they wanted to be. Once I walked in, Kate took me aside.

"I don't know how to say this," she began, "so I'll just come out with it. There's something that happens, something that scares me, and I don't know what to do about it. You see, I thought that our sex life was over. I was fine with that. I thought we both were. But John has become very aggressive about wanting to have sex. Honestly, I don't know how I feel about this. Is it normal? Is his condition—or his medication—making him behave this way? Am I wrong to give in or should I resist? Please, can you help me?"

In another session, this time involving a couple in their 60s, Tom, lean and tanned, who ran a very successful business, told me about his wife Joan who had Alzheimer's. Joan, in a designer outfit and with perfectly coiffed hair and manicured nails, gave off a glamorous air.

"She's been a flirt all our married life, but I was never concerned. I knew it was harmless," he told me, "but now she has become practically predatory, targeting potential sexual conquests wherever she can find them. We went to my 40th college reunion, which I thought was okay because she is mildly sedated. I couldn't believe it; as soon as we got there, Joan was off my arm and sitting in various laps. There was no controlling her. I was beyond embarrassed. I literally had to drag her to our room and lock her in. We left early the next morning. I haven't been able to face my old friends since. More importantly, what am I going to do? How can I help Joan—if she can be helped at all?"

Neither Kate nor Tom understood, much less knew, how to cope with these unexpected sexual behaviors. They did not know that they are a normal part of dementia.

## A NEW REALITY

In my practice as a geriatric neuropsychiatrist, I see patients who are generally 50 years and over. Psychiatric problems in this group tend to involve three general categories—dementia, depression, and delirium—yet almost any psychiatric condition could come my way. Because so many of these problems involve neurological disorders, I also see younger patients who have such diseases, along with Parkinson's disease, stroke, and earlier onset forms of dementia. A good deal of my time is spent leading a 38-bed inpatient service for patient problems that cannot be managed outside a hospital. Particular problems may be medical, such as an acute infection causing a behavior or an end-of-life decision. Other problems might involve social situations, such as intoxication or inappropriate behaviors. Others can be psychological, for instance helping the staff figure out why someone with a personality disorder is acting in a certain way.

However, when I meet men and women whose lives have been touched by dementia, the conversation almost inevitably turns to the very sensitive topic of sex and how it affects them. That circle of conversation ripples beyond spouses and partners. It extends to family, friends, and all kinds of support staff, including medical personnel.

As a physician who has treated over 20,000 elderly patients in the last 10 years, I discuss the subject of sexuality every day, with many people involved in each case.

And while the talk with loved ones naturally focuses on the other worries that dementia brings—is the diagnosis correct, what kind of treatments are available, will long-term care be necessary—it is also predictable that loved ones are blindsided by the development of unexpected sexual behavior. Not only are they unprepared, but they also don't know how to react to it. (They are not alone. Many professional caretakers in adult care facilities, who are used to the sexual actions of patients, aren't taught how to defuse—or permit—these behaviors.) The reason is simple: to date, patients and their partners have been virtually abandoned by an entire medical system that has provided little to help them with sexuality as it relates to dementia. Considering the numbers of people affected—tens of thousands of people in my practice alone—that abandonment is nothing short of shocking.

So it comes as no surprise to me that family members, as well as aides, nurses, and physicians, don't have any good information about the effects of dementia on sexuality. Up until now, there has been little available help, much less explanation, to guide them in understanding unusual sexual behavior or in knowing how to cope with it in dementia patients.

## THE NEED FOR INFORMATION

The popular books and guides about dementia offer a wealth of information but leap past this sensitive subject as though it doesn't exist. And while some discuss the losses and suffering in romantic relationships, they seldom mention sex. This seems odd, since virtually all of those relationships involved sex. Is sexuality such a sensitive subject that it must be hidden away? Have the families been asking the questions about sex and getting little, if any, response? Or do they try to ignore the behavior out of embarrassment or inability to cope with it?

Although sexual-related issues are very commonly seen in dementia—for the person afflicted with dementia, displays of affection are often tied to sexuality—I've observed that family and staff, instead of recognizing what is going on, often deny or actively try to quash the behavior. This, in turn, only alienates the patient more and leads to mistrust, aggression, and even the refusal to take medications and to receive hygienic or nutritional care. In extreme cases, loved ones die.

But in my firsthand experience, I've seen that cases involving sexually inappropriate or unexpected behavior can be helped when everyone involved listens carefully and has a full understanding of the entire situation. Everyone concerned with the patient's care needs to form a unified decision on how to approach the problem, but this is easier said than done. Families may become defensive, caregivers offended, and others, such as the primary care doctors, might just be too busy. Even once the real problem is identified, this group may make few gains at first. Emergency room visits, medications, various behavioral plans, grievances (concerns about the facility brought to the state's attention), patient complaints, and any number of other factors might lie ahead, especially if the behaviors remain difficult and unrelenting.

Nonetheless, the harsh reality is that there are times when sex or expressions of physical intimacy and closeness are the only way that dementia patients have left to communicate with others. This happens frequently in dementia by virtue of the loss of the higher-level cognitive capacities necessary for communication of ideas and feelings. Still, the emotional needs and desires remain inside. The expression of this inner world varies greatly, from subtle gestures to highly inappropriate social behavior.

So the question that has to be answered is this: with all that these patients have lost, or will lose, isn't it cruel to ignore their desire, as well as their partner's needs, for connection and closeness?

## IT'S TIME TO FACE THE OTHER REALITY OF DEMENTIA

*Sexuality and Dementia* is the first comprehensive book to deal with a hidden reality that all too many of us will have to cope with in the future. It is time for the behavior to be brought out into the open and discussed in depth.

To do that, I will explain the physical basis of the connection between sexuality and dementia and suggest ways of dealing with the unexpected behavior that respect both you and your loved one with dementia. For instance, an important effect of illnesses such as Alzheimer's disease is a dramatic change in the habits, customs, and pleasures a couple has gained over the years. These touchstones can disappear while interest in sex, by one or both parties, can continue. There is another effect on long-term relationships: now both partners are faced with strangers. I've witnessed people whose loving companions, now ill, repel them. I've seen men and women who are loyal and faithful to a dementia-affected spouse discover that their partner has fallen in love with another person. And then there are the partners or spouses who yearn to move on emotionally and physically themselves, but don't know when or how to do it, or if it's the right thing to do.

Partners and spouses of patients are not the only people who ask questions about sex and dementia. Staff members in the assisted living and nursing homes I advise frequently seek me out with questions about how to handle patients, as do my fellow physicians and other health care professionals. Given the prevalence of dementia, there is increasing acknowledgment of the sexual challenges that accompany the condition.

Finally, there is interest in finding ways to understand and handle the sexual feelings and actions of men and women who long to connect to others.

## WHAT YOU WILL FIND OUT

The numbers are sobering: About five million Americans currently suffer from Alzheimer's. This number is expected to rise to 20 million by 2050. If other forms of dementia are added, the current number is closer to seven million, rising to 25 million by mid-century. Most of us will, in some way, be affected. With so much at stake, I believe it's time to understand sexuality and dementia and to learn how to deal with it in the most humane ways.

Every person whose spouse, partner, family member, or friend is diagnosed with dementia deserves to know that there are positive ways of dealing with unexpected sexual behavior, such as flirtation, masturbation, verbal abuse, grabbing, and exhibitionism, that accompanies the condition. In these chapters, I will address all the questions I am most frequently asked and include information on the following:

- The fact that when short-term memory vanishes, fundamental behaviors, such as fear, sadness, happiness, and sexuality, are heightened—this is the time when inappropriate sexual behaviors take place;
- The underlying biology and psychology of the different forms of dementia, including age-related Alzheimer's disease, stroke-induced dementia, Parkinson's disease, and Lewy body disease, as well as the causes of dementia seen in younger people;
- An understanding of the relationship between dementia, aging, and sex, and how sexuality is a healthy part of growing older;
- The reality that dementia in general is probably underdiagnosed due to it being relatively low on the medical radar and the family/spouse denial factor;
- The different roles sexuality plays in those with dementia, including one's sense of self and self-confidence;

- The effects of medication (and overmedication), both prescribed and over-the-counter, on sexual behavior;
- The failure of the health care establishment to deal with the challenges related to sex and dementia;
- The management of unexpected conduct;
- An understanding of how emotional connections can be distorted in dementia (for instance, love may become funny and sexual excitement may be accompanied by either sadness or anger);
- The impact of religious and cultural values on decisions made by partners and spouses;
- The personal choices partners can make and how the illness may reshape views of sex and intimacy outside the marriage for both the patient and the partner.

All these points will be illustrated with true stories of patients and their partners to help every person whose life is affected by dementia understand that unexpected or inappropriate sexual behavior and other problems related to sex may arise. I have changed the names and identifying characteristics of all people in these stories so as to protect individual privacy. The events described are normal and happen every day. The stories will show that while many patients are redirected to other forms of closeness, many are able to form some of the most meaningful moments of their relationships.

Those who read this book will become more aware of this sometimes hidden, and yet often blatantly obvious, world of sexuality and dementia. Couples reading this book may notice descriptions that remind them of elements of their own relationships. There is much you will learn of what lies hidden deep inside our partners and ourselves. I hope this will lend itself to a broader understanding and appreciation of the human condition. Armed with this new knowledge, you may even encounter situations where you can make a difference to someone.

Professionals, from caregivers to physicians, after reading this book, may make treatment and management decisions involving both dementia and non-dementia patients with a deeper understanding of our lives as human beings. The result will be a more profound quality of care.

It's time to open the door to the hidden world of sexuality and dementia.

CHAPTER TWO

# Relationships Revisited

Dementia is much more than a disease in which a mind is gradually lost. It is a monumental life event that can severely impact numerous people beyond the patient. No one, however, is more impacted than the romantic partner.

Whether a couple has been together for decades or meet in their later years, a diagnosis of dementia means that the relationship is changed forever. The dynamics of the give-and-take, the negotiations over stress management, and certainly romance itself will never be the same. Behavioral challenges may now routinely occur, when previously they had only been present with stress or intoxication, if at all. The partner with dementia may suffer from unstable moods, loss of social boundaries, or a psychotic reaction to short-term memory loss. These changes are complex and may differ depending upon the type of dementia.

While insight and understanding of the disease varies, it is common for patients to not recognize many symptoms and changes. It could not be more the opposite for the healthy partner who is witnessing firsthand the beginning, middle, and end of a dramatic saga, which might last years. In some ways, dementia is worse for the healthy partner who, in general, will more consciously need to deal with the loss of what was and absorb the responsibility of what now is. This all takes place while the one with dementia is unknowingly drowning in confusion. This partner disparity will only grow as the dementia progresses—and with that will come stress. Nowhere else in the relationship will this stress be more evident than in the most intimate aspects of the partners' lives.

For every intimate relationship, there are two individual psyches that joined together to form a bond based on common interests and compatible personalities. (Perhaps the most basic commonality between two people in a romantic relationship is that both are usually either homosexual or heterosexual.) While many factors play a role in intimacy and romance, some will be affected more than others by dementia. From my experience and observations over the years, the patient can forget how to walk, talk, or even swallow, but the basic sexual orientation tends to stay intact.

On the other hand, the subtleties of love, the sometimes small but noticeable idiosyncrasies or even shortcomings, might quickly vanish. These can be the most devastating of all the losses. To be sure, most couples will have less of a sex life over time, but sexuality seems to be always there, lingering, in one subtle form or another. This is a constant I have witnessed many times in my practice, no matter how the personality of the affected person regresses.

## STEPPING BACKWARD

The regression of dementia is more than just the loss of brain cells, particularly as the condition relates to love for another person. Many partners of dementia patients report that the other person's ability to love and empathize seems to diminish. The relationship regresses to one of more dependency. For some, this comes with paranoia and jealousy in a person who was never that way as an adult. Other patients seem to become a caricature of their previous personality. Those who were once pessimists suddenly become profoundly depressed. Others, who were obsessive, become hoarders, and others might change dramatically in unpredicted ways. Still, most exhibit a loss of any ability to control impulses, along with childlike frustration intolerance. Rather than dealing with an exasperating problem in a rational way, they are more likely to act out with anger, become depressed, or avoid the issue all together.

Unfortunately, beyond the reality that the patient is losing his mind, or getting senile, few doctors address the psychology of the regression of dementia. This is critical to a couple experiencing such a devastating blow. So where do we go to understand more about the psychology of this regression? Can we look to psychological events at other phases of our lives?

Many people observe that dementia patients regress back to a childlike attitude. Jealously and paranoia are two of the most common and pronounced problems faced by couples in which one partner has dementia. But other issues, such as hoarding, and highly dramatic behavior, like anorexia, skin picking, and hairpulling, are seen as well.

Many theories put forward by well-known names in psychoanalysis describe these behaviors as remnants of early stages in our psychological development. Sigmund Freud talked about the three stages of psychosexual development: the oral, anal, and phallic phases. The oral phase, found in young babies, is linked to paranoia and jealousy. Adults who are excessively paranoid and jealous are said to be stuck in this oral phase. Melanie Klein, another renowned Austrian psychoanalyst, found the same linkage in what she called the "paranoid position." Her theories, still debated against the more traditional Freudian ideas, are best known for her idea of the *paranoid and depressive positions*. These are based on the idea that children are the most self-centered and narcissistic beings on the planet. They have little ability to think outside of their own world and thus no ability to think or care about others. Most psychological theorists agree with Freud and Klein that as adults the majority of us work through these early, more primitive, views of the world. We care about others as people rather than just objects that provide for us. According to Freud, later developmental stages may also be connected with other issues, such as obsessions in the anal stage or dramatic histrionic behavior in the phallic phase.

Whether you subscribe to such theories or not, the fact remains that different character descriptors, such as obsessive, narcissistic, and histrionic, have endured as a part of our psychological jargon and everyday language. While we sometimes use the terms jokingly, these personality types may have serious consequences. There is nothing to laugh at when it comes to the compulsive expression of love by someone with an obsessive personality style who gives little else, much less the confusion of a hysterical person who cannot be calmed to ever again talk seriously about love.

Consider Linda. Described as a somewhat obsessive type by her husband Fred, she was fastidious and clean, and their house was always in perfect order. Because Linda had suffered a terrible blow as a child when both her parents were killed in a boating accident, Fred always thought that Linda's perfectionist nature was the result of this tragedy, a way of cleaning the loss away. Whether or not this was the case, this aspect of Linda worsened as she developed Alzheimer's disease in her late 60s. Cleaning turned into obsessive collecting and organizing. She was unable to let anything leave the house, except, sadly, the love between her and Fred. A year after her diagnosis, the relationship was gone. Linda's entire focus was on keeping things, not people.

Then there was Martin, a retired airline pilot who had always been the dominant one in his relationship with Jill. They were married for over 50 years and had several children, all of whom called him Martin because he was away so much. Still, their lives all centered around him—not because he was such a great father and husband but because he always seemed to focus on himself. According to one of his daughters, because Martin was such a strong character, the rest of them just followed his lead. Yet the entire family reported that he always seemed empty when it came time for a one-on-one conversation. It didn't surprise his family that he became very paranoid when his dementia started because he'd always been so grandiose about himself, even while seeming so fragile beneath the surface. Once he became confused, he read into situations and became more than curious about his status and stature with others. He became suspicious of people and especially their motives. Martin's narcissistic behavior was mirrored in his dementia.

If the narcissist seems cool, calm, and certain, the hysteric is just the opposite. While attention and approval is a common aim, the hysteric must continuously create a drama through deception and social manipulation to force his or her status into place. Sandra had only mild dementia at age 62 when suddenly, seemingly out of the blue, she presented severe confusion and Parkinson's symptoms. (Coincidentally, her much older spouse with Parkinson's had recently been placed in a nursing home.) Both of her parents had died of Alzheimer's. She was alone, except for an older sister who was convinced Sandra was faking her symptoms because she had always cried wolf. After interviewing Sandra, we discovered that she used hysterical behavior as a way to connect with people she missed. Pointing out this behavior to Sandra quite dramatically returned her back to her stable and only mildly confused condition.

I mention these three personality types to demonstrate the spectrum of character types. Some are very social and some extremely alone, others are deeply disturbed and still others not so much. A number of people are influenced by constitution, while many are shaped by experience and abuse. I find that one of the interesting things about dementia is the way in which it seems to magnify personalities—the person's childhood, in a way—into a sort of caricature of what they were before. I have seen this many times. Families often report it as well. To be sure, not all narcissists become paranoid and not all obsessives hoard. New personalities can come forth out of nowhere while previous personalities dwindle. It seems to me, though, that without some elements of the past person, exaggerated or not, the patient can more quickly lose sight of a partner, as well as the relationship.

## COMPARING THE PERSONALITY TYPES

When I taught at Columbia University Medical School, I used the following story of three runners in a Central Park race to help med students differentiate three basic personality types.

The hysteric becomes outraged at a person who passes him just because he is being passed, but he owns the emotion and directs it at the right person. Thus, the hysteric is healthier than the obsessive who, when passed by the same guy, gets crazed and looks down at his watch. He also owns the emotion, but it is displaced to the watch, away from what he's really mad at.

The obsessive, in turn, is healthier than the narcissist, who, when he is passed, smiles and shakes his head at the passing runner, certain that the runner sneered at him when passing. He doesn't own his emotion. Instead, he projects the emotion onto the other runner, missing things altogether, and is one step away from paranoia.

Paranoia, based upon the primitive defense mechanism of projection, is common to narcissists and explains why they are so mentally fragile. When one's unconscious feelings are projected, the false belief that the other person is angry (or whatever) feels real. This is just a step away from a belief that the person is, somehow, out to get the narcissist.

These are just three of many "styles" of navigating our world, found in all people, and originating to some degree from birth as well as from life events. It is important again to realize that our personality does not go away in the face of dementia—far from it. The dramatic hysteric, the obsessive hoarder, the narcissistic paranoid psychotic each will have a different course in their disease, in part determined by their personality.

And for the caregiver or partner too, their personality will affect the way in which they approach their challenges. Can you think of the differences in coping skills a hysterical versus obsessive versus narcissistic partner might have? Which do you think would do better?

In addition to the heightened character traits, the loss of executive function, so common to advancing dementia, leaves reasoning by the wayside. Executive function is the ability to plan, reason, and control emotions. This is a function of the frontal lobe, which is usually affected later, after the memory loss occurs in Alzheimer's, which first affects the hippocampus and other memory centers. Some dementias, like Pick's disease or frontotemporal dementia, which occur in younger people, start with frontal lobe disintegration. In those cases, changes in executive function and personality occur before memory loss. (How different types of dementia affect the brain is covered in chapter 3.)

With changes to executive function, patients see everything as either an immediate threat to be gotten rid of or an immediate desire to be fulfilled. For many dementia patients, this may quietly appear as either apathy or a busyness. But the result in relationships is often heavily manifested by such attitudes as frank withdrawal, defensiveness, and jealousy on one hand or excessive sexuality, restless overinvolvement, and a fight for power on the other. A sense of desperation by all involved may soon follow, even to the point of a hostage-like situation within what once was a stable and loving relationship.

And oftentimes, sexual behaviors are deeply integrated into individual identity, security, and power.

## PARANOIA AND THE POWER STRUGGLE

I met Jesse and Rose not long after Jesse was diagnosed with dementia and forced to relinquish his driver's license, the ID people use for most of their lives. "Who am I without my license?" he asked me. Losing the right to drive was just the first in a long line of touchstones that disappeared. He didn't question who he was as much as wonder who he was relative to another person. Jesse asked Rose if she was really his wife, and he wanted to know if they were in Seattle, where they had moved 20 years earlier, or back in Hackensack, New Jersey. A retired oral surgeon, Jesse demanded to know, "Where's my dental chair and my staff and my patients?"

Jesse's attempt to hold onto his personal identity so vehemently was the root of much of his agitation and behavioral problems. With his profound loss of identity, his sense of personal security—especially in his relationship with Rose—vanished. His insecurity turned into paranoia when he began accusing her of having an affair with his best friend. Rose, appalled and angry, pushed back. "I know he's sick," she told me, "but he is endlessly insulting, too. Not only does he keep asking me if we are married, he insists that I'm carrying on with someone else. I can't help myself. I keep being pulled into arguments with him, even though I know there isn't any way to win them."

I explained to Rose that the last thing a dementia patient will admit is a loss of his sense of self. "You can expect insecurity to be at the root of most of the power struggles," I told her. "As the sense of self diminishes, as we see in dementia patients, insecurity grows. With the increasing insecurity comes a sense of powerlessness. Most people won't let power go without a fight."

At this point in the conversation I realized that Rose was feeling as powerless as Jesse because she couldn't help him. I tried to convince her that she could play a huge role in aiding him. We talked about how vulnerable Jesse was inside, and about his paranoia being a part of the regression of his disease, aggravated by his insecurity. She soon realized that she had taken over all of the duties in the household and was regularly disciplining him rather than treating him like a partner, let alone any kind of lover. "He must feel like a child," she realized. Jesse had lost both his driver's license and his romantic license. His response was paranoia and psychosis. Understanding this, Rose took a more passive and less controlling role when it came to sex, which is how they had always been. Eventually, with the aid of medication, Jesse calmed down and began to focus on just them instead of an imagined third party.

This sort of jealous paranoia is a very common dilemma for couples dealing with dementia. It seems to be equally common to men and women. One might think that a couple with a previous history of infidelity or other insecurities would be more vulnerable to it, but my experience tells me that it is just as likely to happen in a previously intact, lasting, and sound marriage. In truth, the best predictor of jealous paranoia is the personality of the affected individual.

While I did not know Jesse before his dementia set in, Rose described his pre-illness personality as "always all about him and self-centered." Thus it would make sense that he would fall apart the way he did because he had a narcissistic type personality.

Dementia's effect on sex and romance will vary from couple to couple, but there will always be an effect, and it will be marked. I saw this played out with Ted and Zoe, a Greek couple I encountered years ago.

## THE DESPERATION OF MISUNDERSTANDING

Ted and Zoe suddenly started fighting, and their children feared that one of them might get hurt as some of these battles escalated to slapping each other and throwing things. The situation was a mess and trying to sort out what was going on through all the "he said, she said" with a couple that was so highly emotionally charged seemed nearly impossible. I recommended that they separate and let things settle down. Zoe seemed particularly devastated by the separation, which seemed odd considering what we were about to discover from Ted. At this point, Zoe hadn't received a formal diagnosis of dementia, but her mild memory issues were apparent to those around her.

After a week or so, in a much calmer state, Ted was able to divulge that he had become upset that Zoe was no longer sexually active with him. He believed she was no longer interested for a variety of reasons: she was angry with him, she was having sex with someone else, and she had lost interest in him entirely. None of this made sense to one daughter who was quite savvy and interested in working through what was really going on. Why would her mother suddenly take issue with her father's dominance? They had always been that way. She was as submissive as he was dominant, and the idea that she would have an affair made no sense at all. In other words, the relationship was based upon her following his lead. How then could she gather up the independence and gumption required to stray from the marriage?

The other daughter, with whom Zoe was now living, gave me another clue. Zoe was experiencing a worsening of her short-term memory and seemed increasingly distressed by her confusion, especially in the afternoon. We knew that she had suffered small strokes over the past few years, but there was no paralysis, which would be typical of a big stroke. (Chapter 6 covers stroke-related dementia in detail.) No one had ever considered that the events might be affecting her mind. Not only was she experiencing the development of stroke-related confusion, she was also presenting another phenomenon typical of stroke disease called pseudo-bulbar affect. With this symptom, emotions run wild, with episodic involuntary outbursts. Inappropriate laughing or crying is typical, but anger may occur as well. This neurologic development, with the confusion, was slowly mixing into the highly dramatic behavior in the household.

Still, Zoe was legitimately upset that she was separated from her husband and desperately wanted to be back with him. This was no woman cheating on her husband. What she was experiencing were frank symptoms of dementia made worse by her separation from familiar situations and environments, and most of all, Ted. Zoe was experiencing environmental regression. The term is used to describe the common but little understood phenomenon of patients becoming more confused from environmental changes. Sometimes the confusion results from a change as simple as a planned move or vacation; at other times it could be provoked by the presence of another person in the house, like a health aid or other caregiver. Something as simple as a change in the weekly visit by a grandchild who has now gone off to college can trigger the regression. Sadly, sometimes the outcome is a by-product of treatment or hospitalization. It is often irreversible.

It seemed that Zoe did, on some level, sense her worsening confusion while with Ted and reacted to it by focusing—even obsessing—on her daily duties such as cooking and cleaning, and becoming a caricature of the good, subservient wife she always had been. While many patients may be initially aware of their short-term memory loss, a point comes where they seem to slip beneath the confusion, unaware of what is really happening to them but nonetheless sensing the possible consequences, such as loss of independence or even the departure of a spouse. No one can know for sure what Zoe was thinking, but it was as though she worried that someone would discover her mind's changes (which were already obvious) and force her to leave the love of her life.

It was ironic that Ted saw things so differently. His understanding of what was going on couldn't have been more off the mark. Sex had only taken a back seat due to her exhaustion and depression over the other factors. With this in mind, Ted and Zoe's daughters and I decided to reunite the couple with more structure and supervision, including in-home assistance with the day-to-day chores. I explained Zoe's dementia to Ted, at which point he feared hurting her by having intimacy. The family and I encouraged it, and things seemed to stabilize from there.

Yet it is not an easy task for many—if not most—to talk openly about sex lives within the family, particularly when it comes to the children addressing parental intimacy. Those families working through the process of dementia in a family member will, however, gradually learn that there will be many previously personal aspects of life that need to come under examination, each of them important to the quality of their loved one's life. This is not the time to be embarrassed, but rather to step up to the task in as respectful and validating a way as possible.

Two people, each responding to the change of dementia, try to express, redress, or suppress their needs as best they can. A sexual relationship is likely the most complex and demanding psychological task that humans encounter, and dementia occurs after most relationships have matured and evolved over years. Suddenly the couple is faced with all the things that would have prevented their relationship from forming in the first place: behaviors like one partner's loss of social inhibitions, distorted emotional connections, confusion, and unstable moods. Inevitably, the short-term memories will fade too.

Yet sometimes the memory of sex together may be all that is left for the person with dementia.

## HOSTAGES TO CHANGE

Bonnie and Dale were married nearly 40 years when Dale developed dementia. Their relationship was solid but romantically had slowly developed into more of a companionship. They had not had sex in years. The turning point came a couple of years into the disease when Bonnie needed to spend some time away—"just to get out and breathe," as she put it. Her life, always home based but now tied to caretaking, had become boring and emotionless. At the same time Dale had begun masturbating regularly, and with less and less awareness of his privacy.

A part-time caretaker, middle-aged, outgoing, and friendly, was brought in to help. She and Dale hit it off immediately. Bonnie took the time to explain her concern about his masturbating and the need to set proper limits. The caretaker seemed experienced enough to understand that the behavior was a symptom of the dementia and felt she could deal with it. Although tentative after years of doing the caretaking herself, Bonnie soon felt comfortable leaving him alone with the caretaker, Marilee, for a few hours each day. Things went well for a while until one afternoon when Marilee, in tears, approached Bonnie after she arrived back home.

Marilee related that Dale had suddenly become sexually aggressive with her. She was able to keep her distance, but he had demanded to masturbate in her presence. It was traumatic, as she could not flee from her role of responsibility and nearly called 911. Marilee said that she no longer felt comfortable with him and terminated her position.

This also traumatized Bonnie. She thought long and hard about what had happened.

A friend told her about a support group that I hold and after the first meeting she approached me. After hearing her story, I suggested to her that perhaps, rather than her boredom at home, it was Dale's "new found" sexuality that was the reason she needed to get away. Bonnie connected with this idea immediately. This was why she had been completely avoiding social contact with Dale. She kept him in a separate room when not tending to basic care needs such as cleaning and eating. She was unable to deal with the brewing sexual behaviors that Dale was exhibiting.

This might have been one of those cases where insight and awareness help a couple reconnect. Sadly, this would not be the case with Dale and Bonnie. Though Bonnie understood that her emotional reactions were healthy, the underlying problem couldn't be solved. She was truly trapped. There was no other family to reach out to. Friends had fled years ago, and the family doctor didn't have a clue about dementia, let alone this sexual nightmare.

Several days after the incident with the caretaker, Dale became extremely agitated after Bonnie refused to have sex with him. The scene was ugly; they were in the street arguing in their pajamas when the police, called by a neighbor, arrived. From there, they went to the emergency room. Bonnie knew that they were only going to tranquilize Dale and send him back home with her. Realizing she had her foot in the "help door," she declined to take him, despite the ER social worker claiming she couldn't do that. "The hell I can't," responded Bonnie angrily.

It took the emergency department staff more than 36 hours and considerable sedating medication to realize that they had a geriatric psychiatric emergency on their hands rather than a case of domestic violence. Finally they referred Dale to my service, where we hospitalized him and looked the situation over. It was clear that Dale suffered with dementia and that there were some dynamics between the couple that were not favorable to Dale's confusion. As his disorder grew, he began to feel helpless and powerless around Bonnie, whose distancing herself had only made it worse. The final straw appeared to be an antidepressant that Dale was put on for his depression and apathy. This had only agitated him further, making him more irritable, hypersexual, and desperate to prove himself in his confused way. Dale's medications were adjusted, but Bonnie was still unwilling to take him home. In the end, we decided that Dale would be best suited for an assisted living facility for dementia care, with a staff trained and skilled in a way that would allow him to have the best quality of life, including social interaction. Could he continue to masturbate in the privacy of his room? Yes.

This case underscores the fact that all relationships are not created equally when it comes to dementia. In terms of each individual, the afflicted person will always portray a great deal of unpredictability. Some, who had been very sexual in nature, will decline in that regard. Others who had been prudish will become sexual savages in the bedroom. One thing is certain: Sex, or the absence thereof, will always be attached to a value or dynamic in the relationship. It is up to the healthy partner to identify that and make the most of it.

It seems clear that the healthy partner will need to be strong in his or her solitude and patient when seeking reward. Sadly, the needs of the healthy partner are not likely to be met as they were before. Nonetheless, I've seen many healthy men and women maintain a desire to learn about the changing dynamics of their partners in order to continue a lasting relationship. Otherwise, the situation will go unattended with no adjustment for the confusion. The partners will become strangers, basically a caregiver and a patient.

## MISTAKEN IDENTITY

Extended families and friends are also affected by the changes that dementia brings. Such was the case with Earl and Sandy. These two, in their mid-70s, had always been active members of a local golf club. They had developed many close and meaningful friendships over the years. As is usual with most cases of dementia, many friends disappeared, yet an extraordinary number of people at the club chose to remain close to the couple as Sandy drifted further and further into her memory loss and confusion. They were treated with the same respect they had always enjoyed. Some friends had more skill and a higher level of comfort than others in deflecting her silly questions or comments, but it was the group effort that they all felt humbled and proud to be a part of. The extra hug and kiss that Sandy would sometimes offer was well received and exerted a positive effect on the group as a whole.

But then problems arose. Sandy slowly became more flirtatious. At first, it all seemed frivolous and immature, with random touching or inappropriate comments to either sex. These things were "just a little out of bounds" as Earl put it, but he could see the rising tension in the others. "They were quieter, more distant," he told me. Earl felt he had to do something. He could see that alcohol, which had always been a part of the social scene at the club, was making Sandy's behavior worse. With the group's help, he began replacing the alcoholic drinks with virgin ones. It was then that Earl realized how far Sandy's dementia had advanced; she didn't even notice the difference. Removing the alcohol did, however, have a positive effect on her. The flirtatious behavior subsided and the numbers of friends around them slowly grew once again. There was a long stretch of time after that where things were status quo—until Earl noticed something else.

Ned was a handsome man in his 70s who was visiting friends of some fellow club members. When Ned returned to his seat at the bar after a brief absence, Earl noticed that he seemed distracted and had a slight smudge of pink lipstick on his lips, as if it had been incompletely wiped off. At first Earl found this amusing and began looking around the room for the woman he could have possibly been with. It was then that he noticed Sandy was missing from his side. He immediately set out on a search, only to find her in the parking lot being redirected by some friends who knew her well. This wandering was not a rare occurrence and Earl thought nothing more of it until he saw that her signature pink lipstick had been smudged. He had no question in his mind as to how that had happened.

Earl was not the jealous type. Despite her condition, sex had actually been strong between him and Sandy, but he knew how vulnerable she was. He asked friends to watch Sandy and returned to the bar to confront Ned. Earl angrily faced Ned just as he was leaving, and was so loud and accusing that several men intervened to prevent a fight. The onlookers gasped as Earl detailed what he thought had happened and the outrage he felt given his wife's dementia. Earl slowed when he noticed the tears in Ned's eyes. Then Ned asked to speak with Earl in private. The two men stepped out onto the lawn.

Ned explained that what had happened was equally upsetting for him. His wife had died of Alzheimer's a few years back. When he rounded the corner coming out of the bathroom Sandy suddenly came upon him and kissed him on the lips. Stunned, he backed away and inquired who she was. Sandy said, "What is the matter with you, Earl?" He had no idea at the time who Earl was. More to the point, he knew the confusion of dementia. He'd thought he was finally letting it go, but it had all come back to him at that moment. He asked his friends to leave because he could no longer stay. Earl could see the honesty in his eyes. The two men cried together, holding one another by the arms and apologizing to each other.

Strange things can happen when sexuality, the ever so socially delicate and yet powerful aspect of who we are, comes into contact with either the confusion of dementia or the bewilderment of someone close not knowing how to respond to it. Sandy and Earl were fortunate; their friends were loyal and understanding. This allowed them to spend more time together and to go on living a similar life to what they had for years until Sandy's care needs became overwhelming.

Yet as much as the symptoms of dementia are similar, each case is unique to the people involved.

## THE PARTNERS' ABYSS

A few years ago, Ken, in tears, shared his anguish over his partner Kyle, who at 48 was struggling with advancing HIV dementia. They had been very much in love through their entire relationship of 20 years and had deeply enjoyed one another romantically and sexually. In their third decade together, Kyle began to drift away emotionally and his personality changed. He became more outgoing, his comments increasingly sharp and witty. He began drinking and going out more. Then came nights when he was literally gone, only to return a day or two later. They might have broken up were it not for the fact that Kyle wound up in an emergency room and was admitted with a manic episode, which was, unfortunately, the early signs of HIV dementia. Kyle was diagnosed with AIDS.

The mania left Kyle almost as soon as it had arrived—in a matter of weeks. For some time he was lucid. It was during this period that he confessed to Ken that he had probably had unprotected sex with 15 to 20 men during the course of his wild manic nights out. If there was ever an opportunity for jealousy, it was then. But that didn't happen. Ken could see that something terrible was happening to his partner. Physically Kyle looked thinner and drawn, but what was most striking was that the person Ken loved was vanishing emotionally, as if the lights of their romance and love were on a dimmer and were slowly being turned off. As is often the case in dementia, Ken pushed on, caring for Kyle while getting nothing in return in the way of emotion. He watched his companion wane over the next two years until dying as a result of the pulmonary complications of AIDS.

Such a story of a slow and gradual fading away from romance is common to many individuals in a relationship with someone who has any sort of dementia. In some ways, this aspect of dementia seems worse than being on the receiving end of anger or aggression, which at least requires some acknowledgment that the partner is there. With or without sexual behaviors, the ability to love back is difficult to sustain.

## NO LOOKING BACK

So what, if anything, is to be gained by taking the time to move forward romantically when the disease is taking the sick partner away from all the years of emotional growth attained together? Part of the answer, once again, is found inside the healthy partner's personality and determination to understand what is happening. For many partners, maintaining the relationship is the only option.

Each partner will have to endure years of progressive changes in the dynamics of the relationship, including the balance of love and power, sexual behavior, and social conduct. For the afflicted one, a slow regression to a more primitive existence in the relationship may mean that sexuality becomes more important as a means of maintaining an identity and a way to grasp glimpses of love. For the healthy partner, conscious adjustments will be necessary for romantic life to go on. Learning to expect less conscious acts of love while searching for more subtle moments will become the norm. Still, hidden in the midst of this tragedy may be unforeseen opportunities, and a brief togetherness that would have otherwise never existed.

No one can tell this story better than a spouse or partner. The subtle and yet insidious changes of dementia are something they struggle with, perhaps even more than the patient. And as if that were not enough, it is up to the partner to make the most of the remaining time together, which may be many years.

Through understanding and a willingness to adapt, you can maintain an emotional connection. I believe it's worth trying to do, as it will improve the quality of your life and that of your partner's, for the time it is possible to do so.

CHAPTER THREE

# The Neurobiology of Sex and Dementia

So much is yet to be understood about the neurobiological relationships that occur between sexuality and dementia. Anxiety and paranoia as a result of memory loss color relationships. Hypersexuality, stemming from a manic storm arising from the surge of certain brain chemicals, puzzles caregivers. Inappropriate behaviors due to loss of inhibition or planning ability confuse and appall family and friends.

Yet, it appears to me that, no matter how much we learn about the brain and the body and how dementia affects them, there will always be an inexplicable sexual connection. Factoring in the person's predisease personality may not prevent the aberrant behavior, but it should steer the attempt to understand it. Personalities can be amplified when something goes wrong in the brain. When that happens, a docile person may become more passive; a dominant individual may become more overbearing; someone who has always been somewhat paranoid may become unrelentingly suspicious, unreasonable, and mistrustful.

However, there are some general things known about the link between neurochemicals (also known as neurotransmitters—they are the chemicals of the nervous system that transmit signals between cells) and personality. For example, higher serotonin levels are associated with social traits and positive moods. Dopamine is connected to thrill seeking, and noradrenaline is associated with aggression and dominance. It's possible that a thrill seeker might seek more sexual excitement as well as take more risk in that direction, or that a giddy social person will stay connected through sex, or that a dominant person's trait might continue to be played out sexually. And while there are many cases where a person withdraws into a state of apathy, essentially losing his or her personality, I have also witnessed the playing out of personality types within the boundary of dementia.

Also, it is important to note that there is a waning of sexual behavior in many cases of dementia, as is true with most neurologic disease. Decreased sexuality is in itself a sexual issue that affects one's ability to reach out intimately. There are two people affected when this happens. Consider the healthy partner on the receiving end of this kind of situation. He or she is losing a physical, as well as an emotional and intellectual relationship.

It is estimated, depending upon the study, that inappropriate sexual behavior occurs in 7 to 25 percent of dementia patients. About a third of those exhibit hypersexual behavior, which means that there is more than just social inappropriateness but an actual increase in sexual desire above the norm for that individual. My estimate, based on my patients and anecdotal evidence from peers, is that the range of problems likely affect over 75 percent of people with dementia.

How can sexuality continue when so much is taken away? For all that sexuality might be normal, dementia could serve as the definition of abnormal. The two seem so opposite that it almost feels wrong to mention them in the same sentence. Nonetheless, they are linked. Understanding how and why they are could make dealing with unexpected behaviors easier.

## WHAT HAPPENS IN THE BRAIN

With so much withering away, why are sexual issues in dementia as common as they are? Few biochemical or neuroanatomic aspects of sexuality and dementia are known, but the answer seems to be in the years before the end stages of the disease. This is when relationships and social functioning are largely intact.

The neurobiological changes of these early and middle years of dementia can have different effects on sexuality. In some cases, normal sexual feelings can be maintained but without the ability to plan or to act appropriately at a social time or place. For others, peripheral symptoms of anxiety or paranoia due to memory loss might affect the ability to perform. In still other cases, there is an actual increase in sexual activity. This could have a variety of causes, ranging from direct neurochemical activation in the brain leading to mania, to desperation to hang onto a lover.

It remains unclear the degree to which these behaviors reflect true hypersexuality, complete with augmented fantasy and drive, or the extent to which they may be a dysfunctional expression of a normal sexual appetite filtered through confusion or disinhibition (loss of inhibition). As a comparison, consider alcohol intoxication: is the "loosening up sexually" a direct response of hypersexuality from alcohol or just a disinhibition of the feelings that are already there?

Little is truly understood about the exact nature of the neurobiologic changes deep in the brain with respect to sexual behavior or the ability to predict it. The goal of this chapter will be to align what is known about the neurobiology of sexuality and dementia with clinical experience and observations.

## THE THREE BASIC SEXUAL PHASES AND THE DEMENTIA EFFECT

Here is what happens in the brain before, during, and after sex, and how dementia affects these phases.

### *Phase One: Libido or Sex Drive*

Glutamate, an excitatory neurotransmitter found in the brain, is the substrate, or building block, for the inhibitory gamma-aminobutyric acid (GABA). This glutamate/GABA interaction is always at play, creating a balance between calm and excitement in the normal brain. It surrounds other processes, such as the sexual drive. Two other naturally occurring substances in our bodies help to create sex drive: (1) dopamine, a neurotransmitter, which is present in the limbic system, the striatum, and the hypothalamus; and (2) testosterone, a hormone present throughout the body but secreted primarily from the testes, ovaries, and adrenal glands.

The limbic system is a complex arrangement of deep brain structures lying on either side of the thalamus. Comprising the hippocampus, the amygdala, the fornix, and the mammillary bodies, the limbic system is involved with memory formation as well as emotions. The hippocampus, which processes short-term memory to long-term and spatial memory, such as remembering surroundings, is critical to the amygdala for proper functioning.

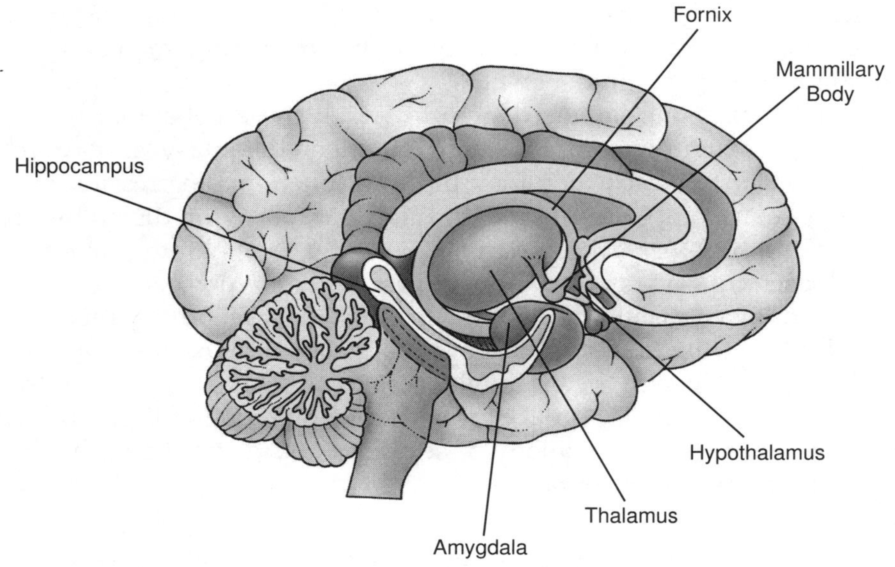


Research has reported the effects of Alzheimer's disease on the integrity of various hypothalamic structures. (The hypothalamus sits just below the thalamus.) These structures are situated between the thalamus and the midbrain. In one study, mention was made of the sexually dimorphic nucleus (SDN) of the preoptic area in the brain and its linkage with sexual drive and orientation. It turns out that this nucleus does not degenerate in the face of Alzheimer's to the same degree as other surrounding structures. The relative preservation of the SDN may explain why a patient's sexual drive is so often preserved.

The two amygdalae lie near the hippocampus and are also involved in processing memory as well as functioning as a primary center for emotion. The hippocampus is connected to the mammillary bodies, two small round masses of gray matter, through the fornix, a bundle of fibers in the brain, where more memories are processed and a connection is made to the hypothalamus. These connections stimulate sexual desire, provide sexual orientation, and function as the primary link from the nervous system to the endocrine system (where hormones originate) through the pituitary gland.

The limbic system also connects with the striatum, a mass of brain matter. Dopamine driven, the striatum serves as a major input center from the cortex. The basal ganglia, a collection of neurons in the striatum, are involved with motor/movement control and are the primary site of destruction in Parkinson's disease through the depletion of dopamine. Another part of the striatum, the nucleus accumbens, is the "pleasure center" involved with addiction, reward, laughter, and fear.

The frontal and temporal lobes, located in the brain's outer cortex, transform memories into a working memory or ability to plan and act rationally, as well as recognize things consciously. The frontal lobes, also highly charged with dopamine, are responsible for conscious decision making, thus allowing for overriding deeper urges in order to avoid inappropriate sex, as well as aggression.

The person you recognize as sexually attractive is greatly determined in the preorbital nucleus in the hypothalamus. The hypothalamus is the connection center between the brain and hormones, which are, in turn, regulated through the pituitary gland.

Sex drive is further enhanced by dopamine, which is the pleasure chemical. Dopamine is closely linked to sexual desire, pleasure, and a sense of reward. (Certain drugs, like cocaine, work by increasing the amounts of dopamine between cells, creating a continuous signal of pleasure. Unfortunately, the feeling runs out, leaving a person with the intense desire to seek the initial feeling of pleasure over and over again.)

**The Dementia Effect:**

- Glutamate increases in those with dementia. In most dementias, it eventually increases to the point of being toxic, causing cell death.
- The hippocampus is a primary target of Alzheimer's.
- Many dementias, in particular frontotemporal dementia, can cause destruction of this part of the brain, leading to serious personality changes, including inappropriate sexual behavior.
- Parkinson's disease, an illness linked to dementia, is the result of a lack of dopamine in the striatum. (Parkinson's-related dementia is covered in chapter 6.) A typical emotional flatness and lack of sexual interest is common. However, a stroke or tumor lesion within the striatum, or even treatment of Parkinson's with excessive dopamine replacement, may have the opposite effect, namely hypersexual behavior, obsessive and compulsive behavior, or mania.
- Lesions in the hypothalamus have been shown to be associated with hypersexual behavior.

- Dopamine levels are severely diminished in cases of Lewy body dementia. (Dementia with Lewy Bodies is discussed in chapter 6.)
- Testosterone, secreted by the testes, ovaries, and adrenal glands, is the sex hormone that most influences sexual desire in both sexes. Testosterone levels are diminished in Alzheimer's patients.
- Lesions in the limbic system are often associated with compulsive behavior, including sexual actions. Overstimulation with dopamine replacement, and the hypersexuality caused by that, is believed to affect the same general area.

### *Phase Two: Arousal (Erection, Lubrication)*

This phase is largely influenced by the neurotransmitter acetylcholine in the brain and nitric oxide peripherally in the genitals. A lot of the epinephrine and norepinephrine (hormones and neurotransmitters, both are also known as adrenaline) influence is held in check here. The reason is that a person cannot function well sexually when anxious or in the fight-or-flight response mode that triggers the release of adrenaline.

Acetylcholine is present in the peripheral nervous system outside the brain and spinal cord. Epinephrine is present in the central nervous system, which comprises the brain and spinal cord.

**The Dementia Effect:**

- Acetylcholine is severely diminished in most dementia cases. The nucleus basalis, which is the center of acetycholine formation, is annihilated in Alzheimer's disease. With a loss of acetylcholine and damage to the nucleus basalis, there is little to keep adrenaline—and arousal—in check.

### *Phase Three: Orgasm*

Noradrenalin, a hormone, is a key factor in achieving orgasm. Prolactin (a hormone produced by the pituitary gland) and serotonin (another neurotransmitter) cause the relaxation and sense of well-being after orgasm.

**The Dementia Effect:**

- The level of noradrenalin is generally diminished in most dementias.
- Levels of prolactin and serotonin are also diminished in people with dementia.

Here's how the three phases come together for a person with dementia. Cell damage, unbalanced neurotransmitters, and changes in hormones may lead to a more active base sex drive or even a normal drive that becomes uninhibited. Deterioration of social controls also takes place. In other words, these occurrences make it easier for some people to become aroused and more difficult to keep that arousal controlled. It must also be kept in mind that for others such changes will diminish sex drive, which is a common aspect to aging in general, including those with dementia. These changes may also make it more difficult to achieve orgasm and feel satisfied after sex. All of this creates a frustrating loop for the person with dementia, and escaping it may be beyond their power.

In my own research, I've noticed a 30 to 50 percent prevalence rate of inappropriate and/or involuntary emotionality in four neurological conditions related to dementia: Alzheimer's disease, stroke, Parkinson's disease, and traumatic brain injury.

***Sexual Behavior and Brain Lesions***

There are many types of dementia, each with a particular type of lesion. Some are global in scale, effecting large or indiscriminate areas of the brain, while others are specialists that target specific areas. What follows is a list of those lesions that are associated with inappropriate, heightened, or peculiar sexual issues that warrant mention. As a reference, it helps to remember that the gray matter is the outer area where the neuron nuclei are located. The white matter is the deeper area where the connection fibers appear.

**Alzheimer's Disease**

Lesion – toxic protein deposition with secondary inflammatory response

Area Affected – cortex, gray matter, particular focus on temporal lobes/hippocampus

Effect on Sexuality – frontal lobe disinhibition, limbic system dysfunction, including possible Klüver–Bucy syndrome (see page 38)

*(continued)*

*Sexual Behavior and Brain Lesions (continued)*

**Vascular (multi-infarct—multiple areas of dead tissue due to stroke) Dementia**

Lesion – strokes
Area Affected – gray or white matter, specific or global
Effect on Sexuality – frontal lobe disinhibition from frontal lobe annihilation, leading to inappropriate behaviors, specific lesions to limbic system, striatum, or hypothalamus; seizures may lead to mania and hypersexuality
(Stroke-related dementia is discussed in chapter 6.)

**Lewy Body Dementia**

Lesion – toxic Lewy body (a type of protein)
Area Affected – gray matter, cortex with special focus on temporal lobes and striatum
Effect on Sexuality – frontal lobe disinhibition leading to inappropriate behaviors, limbic system destruction/ Klüver–Bucy syndrome

**Parkinson's Disease Dementia**

Lesion – toxic Lewy body
Area affected – subcortex specific to striatum
Effect on Sexuality – hypersexuality from excessive dopamine replacement therapy

**Frontotemporal Dementia**

Lesion – a type of protein that stabilizes a transport system between neurons is destroyed
Area Affected – cortex, gray matter specific to frontal lobes, temporal lobe later
Effect on Sexuality – disinhibition leading to inappropriate behaviors

**Traumatic Brain Injury**

Lesion – caused by trauma
Area Affected – anywhere to any degree
Effect on Sexuality – traumatic lesions in frontal lobes cause disinhibition and small lesions in striatum, leading to inappropriate behaviors; hypothalamus or limbic

*(continued)*

*Sexual Behavior and Brain Lesions (continued)*

system lead to inappropriate or bizarre sexual behaviors; secondary seizures may lead to manic hypersexuality

**AIDS Dementia Complex**

Lesion – HIV virus causes area of destructive inflammation
Area Affected – white matter, subcortex
Effect on Sexuality – disinhibition leading to inappropriate behavior; specific opportunistic infections may lead to abnormal sexual behavior

**Alcohol Dementia**

Lesion – toxic effect of ethanol
Area Affected – global
Effect on Sexuality – disinhibition leading to inappropriate behaviors yet with verbal intelligence preserved, allowing for engagement in social activities

**Huntington's Disease**

Lesion – genetic disorder marked by abnormal protein accumulation in cells
Area Affected – striatum initially; eventually affecting the entire brain through the mutation of an important interactive protein
Effect on Sexuality – compulsive sexual behavior from striatal destruction

**Wilson's Disease**

Lesion – genetic disorder marked by abnormal copper deposits in brain tissues
Area Affected – frontal cortex and striatum
Effect on Sexuality – disinhibition leading to inappropriate behaviors and compulsive sex from striatal lesions

**Creutzfeldt–Jakob Disease (Mad Cow Disease)**

Lesion – transmissible protein called a prion destroys tissue, causing spongiform holes in the brain
Area Affected – global
Effect on Sexuality – disinhibition leading to inappropriate behavior, possibly transmitted sexually to others

## NEUROTRANSMITTERS AND THE DEMENTIA EFFECT

Sexual function requires a lot of systems to work together, and the nervous system plays a particularly important role. The nervous system is a collection of neurons found throughout our body. Capable of transmitting electrically charged messages down their length, neurons induce motor control of muscles, sensations, thought, and emotions. It is this network of the more than 100 billion neurons working together that allows the many complex tasks this system performs.

Neurotransmitters, basically chemical messengers, transmit signals through the small spaces between neurons called synapses. It is in the synapse that the true function of each neuron is determined. This all depends upon which neurotransmitters are released from the end of one cell, which receptors are available at the beginning of the next cell, and what electrical charges are available to turn things on or off after the message is delivered. The changes in the electrical charge in cell layers create an action or a mood. Most psychiatric medications, as well as many other drugs, perform their actions by affecting the functions of neurotransmitters.

More than 50 known neurotransmitters are found throughout the body and come from a variety of sources. Serotonin, for example, is secreted in the gut but also from a specific nucleus in the brain called the raphe nucleus.

**The Dementia Effect:**

- In addition to the lessening of neurotransmitters, dementia patients experience a diminishing of control in certain areas of the brain that contain deep memory processing centers.

## THE BASIC CATEGORIES OF ABNORMAL SEXUAL BEHAVIOR

The categories of abnormal sexual behavior include:

- Relationship issues, such as anxiety, paranoia, or memory loss
- Inappropriate behavior (normal sexual activity but abnormal behavior for the situation)
- Hypersexual behavior

There are many different situations where either inappropriate or even hypersexual behavior might occur in the face of dementia. The following four examples are prevalent in my practice.

### *Memory and Anxiety*

Bill was about to retire as an engineer from a world-class aerospace company when his wife Jen began to notice his heart palpitations after sex. He had a full cardiologic investigation and was found to be healthy. The palpitations continued but still seemed only to occur with sex. On further investigation, his primary physician observed that Bill was more on edge and anxious about having sex. This was odd to Jen, as they had always had such a comfortable relationship when it came to sex. An interesting aspect of this that caught the eye of my colleague, who was involved in the case, was Bill's quiet nature—despite the fact that he was the one with the problem. Intelligent people usually present with an involved explanation of what's going on with them. People with early cognitive problems often quietly hide their confusion.

My colleague recognized that something was going on. Had Bill been 40 years old, she might have suspected an affair or some other issue, but at 76, the three Ds— depression, delirium, or dementia—were entertained first. In the end, there was little to support a diagnosis of depression, and there were no medications or medical problems to support medical confusion or delirium. Then a CAT scan revealed a series of microscopic strokes that developed over time, possibly the result of years of Bill's pent-up anxiety and hypertension.

Finally my colleague determined what was wrong. She put together that Bill was experiencing breakthrough anxiety caused by a combination of general social anxiety, early memory loss, and the adrenaline release during sexual arousal. Bill was given a beta-blocker to calm the effects of the adrenaline, and he did much better. Interestingly (and I feel appropriately), my colleague downplayed the likely vascular dementia diagnosis, which would have thrown Bill into a tailspin. She instead focused on the quality of the relationship while privately counseling Jen about the memory loss. Jen was grateful that my colleague handled it that way.

Trying to understand any behavior, including sexual ones, in dementia patients, often comes down to a judgment call. After delirium has been ruled out, one is left pondering over the dementia itself: Is it the broad brush of the memory loss and confusion that is causing the behavior (paranoia, sexual activity, or depression)? Or is it something more exact, like a specific lesion in a specific spot causing the particular behavior? It is likely a mix of the two.

In Bill's case, his relationship issues were based on anxiety.

### *Frontal Lobe Disinhibition*

The police found Katie, a 38-year-old woman, having sex with a homeless man in Central Park in broad daylight.

The officers recognized her confusion and brought her to our New York City emergency department. She was indeed confused, as well as in a disheveled condition. Thin and malnourished, she lacked identification and could not tell us anything about herself. OB-GYN consultants determined she had likely engaged in aggressive sex multiple times in the recent past. She was cooperative but noted to be socially inappropriate, as she frequently propositioned the male staff in the hospital. I admitted her to my service in psychiatry; she was one of my first patients as a new attending doctor. I diagnosed her with a cocaine psychosis due to the presentation and cocaine in her urine test, and I guessed she was a homeless person. I couldn't have been more wrong.

Things began to turn bad for my diagnosis when, after two days, she remained confused and inappropriate. Then an astute social work intern identified her on a missing person list as the absent daughter-in-law of a well-known East Coast society couple. She and her husband lived a privileged life in New York City. I met her family within hours in a conference room and said little about my initial impressions. By then I had the results of the CAT scan of her brain. Unfortunately, what I had to tell them made me wish that my initial assessment of her had been correct.

Katie's frontal lobes were markedly shrunken. Knowing that this couldn't have happened overnight, I queried them about signs of neurological deterioration. The parents-in-law hadn't seen her in some time, due to an extended vacation abroad. The husband reported his wife's substantial withdrawal and apathy for months, but he too had been away frequently due to his work. He thought she was depressed, and they had argued many times about her going to seek help. Then she disappeared. At this point, I was certain that Katie suffered from a behavioral variant of frontotemporal dementia.

One of the primary duties of the frontal lobe is the executive function. This gives us the ability to plan and anticipate consequences and to override more rudimentary desires and thoughts in order to behave in a socially acceptable manner. It's not hard to imagine, then, that lesions or deficits in the frontal lobes of the brain might lead to problems with executive function as symptoms. Such troubles can be the result of many types of diseases. Tumors, strokes, and trauma are not rare visitors to the frontal lobes. Even Alzheimer's disease, to some extent, may affect the frontal lobes of the brain. But only frontotemporal dementia is specific to the frontal and, to some degree, the temporal lobes of the brain. The disease is considered a presenile dementia because it generally starts before age 65. There is no known cause or cure. Few patients survive more than 10 years.

### *Stroke-Related Mania*

Howard was a 61-year-old successful attorney with no history of mental illness. He was married to a younger woman in her 40s who was an engineer, and they had two teenage daughters. A workaholic, he never took care of himself, ate unhealthily, and had poorly controlled high blood pressure. No one, including his wife, was surprised when Howard suffered a massive stroke that left him partially paralyzed. He soon became very depressed. Over the phone, the wife reported that he had been experiencing some memory problems that had been affecting his work and causing even more stress for up to a year before the stroke. And then, before I saw him, he had an episode of loss of consciousness and was admitted to the hospital. A CAT scan of his brain revealed multiple strokes on the thalamic area that explained all the symptoms he exhibited, including the likelihood of vascular dementia.

After a day or so, Howard awoke as a different person. Not only was he no longer depressed, he was extremely manic. He was elated, loud, sleepless, hyper-religious, and hypersexual, as well flirtatious and verbally inappropriate with virtually all the female staff. This behavior was a great embarrassment to his wife and their daughters. To combat his actions, he was treated aggressively with antipsychotics and mood stabilizers. It took over a month to get his manic symptoms under control, but he was finally ready to be released to a rehabilitation center for continued care. Unfortunately, the sexual symptoms created a great hindrance to his treatment and the ability to get the rehabilitation that he desperately needed because no facility would take him. He was not able to work as an attorney again due to his dementia.

Hypersexual behavior and thinking is commonly a part of mania. While typical of bipolar mood disorder, this illness does not usually begin in the elderly, and new onset mania in such patients is more likely due to a medical problem. Medications, such as steroids, antidepressants, and others, are common causes. Infections, tumors, and seizures are other possibilities, but certainly strokes need to be on the list as they are almost always associated with at least one mood disorder, namely depression. Howard's mania was likely due to the multiple strokes.

### *Klüver–Bucy Syndrome*

Characterized by a diminished fear response, a visual agnosia (inability to recognize objects), hyperorality (an abnormal use of the mouth to examine things, continuous eating or even chewing and biting non-food items), and hypersexuality, Klüver–Bucy Syndrome may be caused by a bilateral (both sides) dysfunction of the amygdala. Typically, this problem is seen in people who have suffered brain infections, such as herpes encephalitis, trauma, or multiple strokes. It may also occur in some variants of Alzheimer's disease through the formation of beta amyloid plaques (an excess of proteins) in the hippocampus or even in the amygdala directly.

It is known that the hippocampus is devastated early on in classic Alzheimer's disease. Given the influence that the hippocampus is thought to exert on the amygdala, and the symptoms seen in many patients with Alzheimer's of hypersexuality, hyperorality, and docility, Klüver–Bucy seems a likely scenario. And if the amygdala is directly affected in more cases of Alzheimer's disease than previously thought, as researchers have suggested, then it is even more likely that Klüver–Bucy is a possibility in those patients. A patient named May, who had Alzheimer's disease, led me to question whether this link existed.

May was a typical long-term care patient in an assisted living facility. As with many patients, over the years she had become more confused and required additional care. By the time she turned 80, she was no longer able to walk or dress herself. Yet she could carry on a lively conversation that progressively involved more and more sexualized content and fearlessness. She eventually became quite intrusive, rolling her wheelchair into men's rooms and announcing her desire for sex. She had to be medicated and to some degree isolated to protect her from others. At the same time, she had another problem we needed to address. She was clearly hyperoral, chewing and biting on everything, including her own arms and fingers. We finally had to use distasteful scents on and padding over her skin to prevent injury. These two problematic behaviors—the sexual and oral symptoms, along with her inability to visually recognize objects—are the three common identifying features of Klüver–Bucy syndrome.

## MEN VERSUS WOMEN

May's case brings up another interesting issue as well. While I feel there is a good chance that changes in her limbic system led to her changed sexual stance, there are other factors that cloud the picture. What if May were a man? Would we still be talking about her limbic system, or more about disinhibition of a "male drive"? And what is the difference between actual heightened sexual behavior and just inappropriate sexual behavior?

There is a trend toward studies that often find that Alzheimer's disease is more common in women. This may, in part, be due to the fact that there are more old women than men. But taking the numbers into consideration, the disease, in some studies, occurs more often and is more aggressive in women. Other studies found no difference between the sexes in any type of dementia, including Alzheimer's.

Another study that reported hypersexual behavior to occur in 2 to 17 percent of dementia patients also showed that the behavior tends to be equally distributed between the sexes. However, the line between hypersexual behavior and inappropriate sexual behavior is fine and seems to vary in definition between the studies. For example, "social impropriety" was found to be higher in demented men compared with women in one study, and another reported a drastically higher incidence of "sexually abnormal behavior" in men with dementia compared to women (93 percent versus 7 percent). These latter studies are much more in line with common views on sex and dementia (i.e., the "dirty old man" syndrome).

In my view, unexpected sexual behavior is related to a variety of factors. For one, there is likely some truth that men are more apt to view the world from a physical/sexual perspective and therefore be more likely to make sexual comments or gestures, which are not necessarily hypersexual. This may be determined by both society and biology. Also, most men are bigger than women, making for more of a threat when presenting with any kind of inappropriate behavior. And most caregivers are women and possibly more likely to feel threatened by men rather than by women presenting with sexual behavior. Thus, male inappropriate behavior is likely to be reported more often.

However, with dementia, the differences between men and women will fade as the disease progresses. While our true sexual orientation—that with which we were born—and images that people have regarding our sexual differences seem to be preserved throughout the course of dementia, inevitably, the end stages of brain deterioration begin to take their toll. Merely eating normally, walking, or having rational thoughts are no longer possible.

## A PATH FORWARD

Given that dementia is ultimately a fatal neurologic disease, eventually there will be no sexual behavior. The destruction of brain tissues, regardless of the type of dementia, will lead to the diminishing of any number of human behaviors, including sexuality. But until that moment comes, it is, I believe, important to understand and respect the sexual needs of every person afflicted with dementia. In no situation will that be more important than for those who are in a romantic relationship. As we shall find, it is ultimately going to be up to the healthy partner to keep an open mind and eye toward changes that might be coming his or her way. Unlike many other illnesses, the diagnosis and treatment are only a fraction of what a couple is up against. Yet when it comes to dementia and romance, there might even be some room for hope.

CHAPTER FOUR

# Unexpected Bonds

One of the most intriguing aspects of my work involves seeing how different relationships can form when dementia strikes. It's also one of the most difficult problems encountered by those men and women who are married to, or partners of, a person with dementia. Who, after all, wonders how he or she would react to the incurable illness of a loved one, which likely will last for years? And even if there is some consideration, how can anyone anticipate the range of emotions? I have seen, over and over again, that a person does not know how he or she will respond to a devastating health situation until it occurs.

Who plans for these situations to happen? Certainly, couples often talk about senility during the course of their relationships, but it is more in the context of placing or not placing someone in a nursing home rather than how one might actually behave when the romance is mangled by dementia.

Dementia forces the kinds of wrenching emotional decisions that few of us would be glad to take on. The choices often alter lives in unexpected ways, with family, societal, and personal pressures playing a huge role. Seeking advice, support, and solace, partners often hear opinions that may hurt more than help. Finding oneself shunned from others who had otherwise been close and understanding can be frustrating. At the same time, receiving support when it is not expected can alter the definition of family and friendship.

In each case of romance affected by dementia, reaction ripples out in an unpredictable social-emotional pattern. It starts with the lover, spreads to the family and friends, and eventually touches acquaintances. In many instances, clergy is involved as well. While some individuals feel empathy, others cast blame. Maybe all that can be said is that for most people involved there is some truth unearthed that only a disease like dementia could find. That truth could be about how they feel about dementia, the reaction of others to it, or the situation they find themselves in.

The personal choices partners can make, and how the illness may reshape views of sex and intimacy for both people, is something that is rarely discussed outside of family, friends, and clergy.

How do people cope with these unique circumstances?

## THE GROUP SHARES ITS PAIN

Every Friday I conduct a one-hour meeting for families and partners in the inpatient behavioral wellness unit where I serve as medical director. All these people are there to get information about their loved ones so that they can act responsibly in making informed medical decisions for them. This is particularly so for the patients on the memory wellness unit, who are too confused to make choices for themselves.

We usually go around the room, giving time to each of the four or five patient representatives who show up. While many of the children of patients—or spouses of shorter-term relationships—are emotionally engaged, the older, longer-term spouses are devastated.

It may be hard to believe, but I have been told, time and again, that healthy, long-term partners still want to continue to be physically close to their afflicted partners. Yet the ill partners often reject them. Many spouses—if not most—who have been married for a long time fit into this category.

It's only a few minutes into their story before they tear up and reach for a tissue. These people would sooner die than slow down their love and commitment. They all made the same promise: they would never leave a loved one alone; they would never put a husband or wife in a nursing home. And so there they are, every Friday, fighting for a role in the discharge planning, always erring on the side of taking their lover back home when the partner is more "manageable." These are the same people who may have beat them up a week before, just for getting a kiss on the cheek.

During that group meeting, I don't hear about the rest of the reasons for being hit or clawed or ignored. Sometimes it's too painful or personal or there's not enough time. But no matter what happens, the level of commitment goes far beyond cleaning or feeding someone. Forty, fifty, or sixty years of romance don't just fade away. The great tragedy of this dedication is that, due to the dementia, it's often one sided.

For instance, there was Donna, a once vibrant woman who, when she was stricken with dementia, disappeared emotionally. She was not at all interested in sex or even being affectionate with Mark, her husband of 42 years. He was shattered. It took Mark a while to speak to the group, but when he did, his emotions were as raw as the marks on his face from a recent attack from Donna.

"You have to understand that she is the only woman in my life," he began. "We were high school sweethearts and didn't have sex until we got married. Like everyone else, we had our ups and downs, but our marriage was rock solid. Now she has slipped away and I am lost. There is no one else for me."

Mark is younger than many spouses I see. He was an engineer with an airline, while Donna had committed herself to their two girls. He worked in the buyer support section of the aircraft manufacturing company. Any time there was a plane stuck somewhere in the world, his team would be called out to get it airworthy, on a runway, and in the air. Mark related how Donna would miss him on his trips but also dream of one day being there with him. Mark was going to show Donna the world. As much as they loved their daughters, the couple became more excited as the girls finished high school.

Unfortunately, it was not to be. Donna was diagnosed with Alzheimer's disease at age 50, just when their younger daughter was about to enter college as a freshman. Four years later, both parents missed their daughter's graduation due to an extreme panic attack Donna had on the car ride there. Donna was so confused and frazzled at the hospital that she didn't remember where they were going in the first place.

Over the next six years, Mark kept the relationship going as best he could. He shared that making love was the only way they had left to connect with one another. Finally, she was admitted to our memory wellness unit after trying to stab Mark with a kitchen knife. He had tried to hug her and she lashed out, smashing dishes and screaming so loud the neighbors called the police.

"When the officers arrived they initially wanted to arrest her for domestic violence," he shared with the group. "I explained that she was a victim of dementia. As I was doing so I had a terrible realization: we were both victims. I feel terrible thinking of myself that way, given what Donna is going through. But it is true, isn't it?"

In response, the others in the group nodded in agreement.

"But even with everything that is going on, I still want to take her home. I don't want to let her go. She's my girl."

His two daughters, who also attended the group, told him it was time to say goodbye to that phase of their life. I agreed with them, and Mark tentatively agreed to a trial of assisted living. Nonetheless, he took Donna back home another two times until he could take no more. They never had that time together in retirement, and Mark will carry the heavy baggage of this loss for the rest of his life.

***Planning for the Future***

Once dementia has arrived, take a deep breath and exhale. It will be a process that will unfold over time. There are, however, practical steps that you can take that will help. They are:

- Take control. Get qualified health care, speak to social workers, and seek financial advice from qualified professionals.
- Allow trusted family and friends into your circle. You need them now.
- Listen to their advice before making any decision.

A couple named Sam and Camille shared another effect of dementia on families. They had taken in his mother, Esperanza, a conservative, quiet, and very religious woman who had become less and less able to care for herself due to memory loss. Esperanza was a simple woman who had lived alone for years, since the death of Sam's father from bladder cancer. It all seemed straightforward. Semiretired, Sam and Camille had time to spend with Esperanza, and she could find privacy in the spare room in their small rambler house. All three had gotten along well over the years.

I was very curious to find out where this story was going, since Esperanza was on our unit. Only a couple months after moving in with them, she was admitted for aggression and violence.

"We are a very close couple, and we enjoy our 'private time,'" Camille began. "We don't have any children, so it was never necessary to gauge how much noise we made in our room. So before Esperanza moved in, we tested it by Sam going down to what would be Esperanza's room while I made 'sounds' back in our room. Then we did the same with Sam standing in the hallway. As you would expect, the sounds were louder. We figured that Esperanza would get up to use the bathroom during the night, so the plan was to put our relations on hold for a bit.

"Things started out fine. I took my mother-in law to lunch and to get our nails done, and we got along, as always. Sam worked on some minor construction in her room, including mounting a large crucifix above her bed and a bigger photograph of Jesus on the opposite wall.

"About the third or fourth night, while watching the nightly news in bed, we heard Mom walking out of her room, down the hall to the bathroom, and back. There was no toilet flush or running water, just a brief delay in the bathroom and then the return trip to the bedroom. This happened several times during the night for a couple of weeks. Neither Sam nor I slept well."

"Of course we asked her about the trips," Sam interjected, "but she said she was fine, and she didn't recall the bathroom trips. We thought it was sundowning behavior and it seemed innocent enough. The bigger problem was that Camille and I were exhausted from lack of sleep. Plus, we were getting very irritable because our sex life was on hold. We started to argue: Camille said that maybe moving Esperanza in wasn't the best idea. But we both realized that what we needed—in addition to a full night's sleep—was time alone. Unfortunately, there was no way we could leave her with anyone. So we came up with the plan to take advantage of my mother's nighttime jaunts since they gave us a clear indication of where she was. When the bedroom door closed, we knew we were clear to make love until we heard it open again."

"I know it sounds a little ridiculous," Camille continued, "but this actually helped for a brief spell until Esperanza began to change her attitude toward me. What was once a friendly manner now seemed territorial and critical. In particular, any overt sign of affection between Sam and me set her off, and she began to attack me verbally. Also, the night trips seemed more frequent, which meant less 'private time' for us.

"But then things really spun out of control. The night before we were going to take Esperanza to the doctor to try to figure out what was going on with her, something new happened. Esperanza clicked off the hall light and shut her door for the third time, which was usually the end of her night walks for a while. We began making love, and I should stress that our door was always unlocked. Minutes later I noticed a dark shadow next to the bed. It was Esperanza, who screamed out the name of her dead husband. She pushed Sam aside and attacked me, scratching me with her long fingernails. It took a long time to get her subdued, and both Sam and I were very shaken by the experience."

At this point, one woman asked Camille if that had changed her opinion of her mother-in-law. "Of course not," she exclaimed. "She is my family."

Despite that commitment, over time the couple came to realize they were not able to provide the full attention and structure that Esperanza required. At the same time, it was important for Sam and Camille to continue their close relationship and stay healthy together so they could be there for Esperanza. They sought treatment for her and it worked. She was treated successfully for a psychosis related to her dementia and discharged to an adult family home with five other women. There she stays, happy and without medication.

***The Decision to Give Care at Home***

Most dementia care takes place at home. There are positive reasons for doing this. For one, this is often a cost-effective way to go. For another, most people want to remain with family. However, if you decide to keep your loved one at home, it is crucial that you be aware of the following:

- Care issues, behavioral and otherwise, will worsen.
- Monitor yourself for burnout or an untenable situation. You are of no use to your loved one if you are perpetually angry and/or depressed.
- Do not accept that either mental or physical abuse directed at you is acceptable.
- When the time comes for a change, remember that you are following doctor's orders. Your health matters, too.

## MIXED-UP MESSAGES

Partners are constantly trying to understand each other in relationships. What does the other person need? What can best provide for those needs, emotionally and physically? What are the motivations for their actions? Answering these questions becomes increasingly difficult when one person has dementia. Lou and Cindy's experience highlights how important it is to seek outside help for a new perspective on the situation. Oftentimes, after years of a pattern, even if intimacy has been good, a shift by virtue of the confusion of dementia may be a challenge for even the most seasoned couples. When nonverbal communication and intimacy begin to replace talking through concerns and working through emotions on a more cognitive level, a new point-of-view to help understand the situation can prove invaluable.

Lou, a jeweler, struggled with stroke-related dementia complicated by aphasia, the inability to speak. In addition to not being able to express his feelings verbally, he was also embarrassed about the partial paralysis of his right arm. Cindy told me that he would hide it under a blanket when people were around.

"I'll be honest with you," Cindy said to the group. "The sex is fine—it's his confusion that turns me off. Last week my sisters came to visit, and Lou wandered in and put his hands on me in a very inappropriate way. Look, I'm no prude, but there is a time and place for everything. The way he is now, it's like there is no sense of either one. I didn't mean to hurt him, but when he acted out I pushed him away."

As a result of her action, Lou fell and suffered a hip fracture. He was later transferred to our service for further stabilization due to depression; it was so severe that he wasn't eating.

One of the other group members suggested to Cindy that perhaps the fall was inevitable, a sort of metaphor for where the lopsided relationship was. Perhaps the point had come for a tough question to be asked: Did Cindy *want* to live with Lou anymore? This woman even cited her own situation; it took her a year before she decided that she wasn't going to put up with her husband's aggression any longer.

Cindy suddenly became very defensive and irritated, lecturing the woman on the difference between aggression and sexuality. This led quickly to more anger and then tears. But then something happened. Looking at the members of the group, Cindy blurted out, "Oh no. He's been trying to reach out to me for love—more and more as his confusion got worse—and all I did was push him away because I was embarrassed in front of my family. Of course my Lou is coming back home with me."

And that is what happened. Lou was discharged with in-home care. Cindy accepted an offer from a social worker to consider our intensive outpatient program designed for higher functioning people to further work through issues such as hers. She had the insurance coverage and the time, given that she now had home care for Lou.

Cindy attended the program two times a week for several months. She interacted with others and even went on medication after recognizing she was depressed. "Losing my man of 45 years is as terrifying for me as this must be for him," she said in another meeting. "Now I see that we just express it differently."

Eventually Lou and Cindy were able to adapt to their communication challenges, realizing that sex for them was now playing a bigger role as a substitute for things like talking. Cindy still preferred that he not be demonstrative in front of her sisters. Now that there was plenty of romance elsewhere, Lou seemed to agree.

As demonstrated above, it would have been difficult for Cindy to recognize what was happening between her and Lou without the unfortunate incident of his hip fracture. Sadly, few people realize ahead of time that there may be new insights about the changing relationship awaiting them. They don't anticipate that patience and persistence are required to allow for an understanding of the changed dynamics between a couple dealing with dementia. Obviously, the characteristics of the healthy partner, including stress coping skills and patience, will have a huge impact on the acceptance of change, and with that, important decisions such as remaining together or not.

Cindy also recognized the importance of taking care of herself as an integral part of this process. Depression and anxiety problems are to be expected in all such situations, and should even be treated if severe enough. They should also be considered a normal sign of the need for a change. Unfortunately, too many partners quickly jump to the "old way or the highway" conclusion, which only inspires more stress or guilt if a separation ensues. Cindy found that by opening up the situation to others, she was able to ease tensions and move the relationship forward in a new healthy direction. Thank goodness we were there to help. Sadly, there are few similar services available across the country to provide such a platform for families to work through these issues. The results are often catastrophic.

## A SURPRISING DEVELOPMENT

Of all the situations that can develop with a couple when dementia is present, the switch to a homosexual preference is perhaps the most startling.

Regressing back to sexual situations in the past by virtue of structural and neurochemical deterioration is a well-known phenomenon in dementia patients. There have even been reported cases of dementia in which the progressive memory loss essentially revealed someone to be homosexual. I have personally seen this more than once, but I have not seen the reverse, that is, a gay person becoming straight.

One case I remember was that of a couple married for 50 years. Peter had dementia and was in the hospital for agitation. His wife, Joan, had been astounded to hear reports from his previous facility that he had been sexually interested in men. She reported that he had never had any gay inclinations. Then, a couple of days after his admission with us, it started anew. Peter tried to make out with his roommate.

After a period of trying to figure out what was going on with Peter, it was concluded that he wasn't overdriven sexually but was just expressing, in his confused way, what was inside of him and possibly held in check for years. Ironically, his dementia may have been therapeutic for him in lessening his anxieties over "coming out." We'll never know for sure.

What I did know though, was that his wife was an understanding and somewhat comical sort who had been "around the block" with her husband's dementia for several years. She seemed to take it all in stride, but I knew other partners who might not. Inevitably, dementia leads families, partners, and caregivers down a path of truth rather than deception, no matter how painful.

## UNTIL DEATH DO US PART?

At other times healthy partners will form—or want to find—relationships outside their commitments and will grapple with societal and religious pressures and guilt. That was a story I heard from two people in the group, Howard and Claire

"'You promised, in front of a church full of people, to stay with Martha through sickness and health, to love and obey. That's your commitment. If you don't honor your promise, you are betraying God as well as your wife. You just can't love someone else because your wife is not the woman you married.' Those were the stark words that my sister-in-law Jean said to me when I tried to talk about my feelings toward another woman," Howard shared with the group. "I don't want to love anyone but Martha," he continued. "But Jean was right. Martha is not the same woman I married. I see her deteriorating and it's killing me. Laura, the woman I met, is someone I can talk to—share a meal with. Laura and I go to a movie for a couple of hours and I put my misery on hold. She helps to lift the burden for a while, and for that, among other reasons, I am increasingly fond of her. I wonder: Is it wrong? Martha and I used to kid that as soon as one of us died, the other should find someone else right away—just as long as the person wasn't as smart and good-looking as we were. But we never talked about what would happen if one of us lost our mind. Why would we?"

But because Howard's guilt was such a heavy burden, he stopped seeing the woman he liked. His family played a very strong role in his decision. As he confided to the group, "I can't fight my sister-in-law, my children, and my minister. It's me against all of them, and it's too much to handle. I'd rather seem contrite and have them leave me be than try to forge another relationship. I don't believe it's fair to me, the woman I've been seeing, or even Martha. If I felt stronger about my options, than perhaps, on some deep level, Martha could pick that up. But I give up."

Claire, a high school teacher, experienced a totally different outcome. She dealt with her own set of heartbreaking circumstances in what was, for her, a very unexpected way. When Robert, her partner—they never felt the need to marry—of 25 years, became too confused to connect with her emotionally after seven years of progressing in his dementia, she made a decision. "I will always love Robert, but I still desire a physical and emotional outlet," she stated.

Facing her own needs, she spoke with friends and family as well as clergy about what she could do. Weighing the answers, and being honest with herself, Claire's decision to move on with another partner both made and lost her friends and altered her relationship with several family members.

"It's not fair, it's just not fair," Claire repeated to me each time she would come to visit Robert or participated in the Friday meetings. In their early 60s, she was healthy and he was suffering with advancing dementia. He had no idea who she was anymore. She was vibrant and strong. I could see from the pain in her face that this disease had changed her life as much as it had altered Robert's.

Robert had been admitted to the unit for depression, something commonly seen in confused dementia patients. But I thought that his mood issues from day one weren't very severe, and I wondered why she had pressed so hard to get him admitted. I told her he would likely be stabilized quickly.

Yet she seemed so frazzled, like someone to whom this was new or who had been through a severe crisis. I couldn't figure her out and wondered if there wasn't something else going on.

As it happened, Robert's hospitalization was relatively uneventful, but then Claire transferred him to a dementia care facility rather than return him to the adult family home. I wondered why.

In general, the adult family home had seemed to be working out fine. Again, Claire had seemed unrealistically concerned that he wasn't receiving good enough care and that was why he was depressed.

It was at the new facility, where I consulted, that I ran into Claire, accompanied by a girlfriend, a few weeks later. She seemed calmer but had a story to tell. So the three of us sat on the beds in an empty room and talked. It was clear that the friend, who put her arm around Claire, was her emotional anchor. "You've got to talk about this," the friend said.

Claire started the discussion by stating, "I'm so pleased now that Robert is in better hands. But I keep wondering: Do you think there is any chance of him improving to the point where he could come home?"

Her question perplexed me; Claire knew that Robert's prognosis was clear: He was never going to recover any of his lost faculties. Then, Claire put everything into focus.

"I must be sure that he never will get better because there is so much I need to take care of on my own. I still work and keep my checkbook balanced, but Robert paid the bills and oversaw our investments. He planned trips and loved dealing with the smallest details, something I can't stand to do. And now that I'm seeing Phillip, I want to focus on him while still making sure that Robert is being taken care of. Besides, my family relies on me to be there for them, too."

"Hold on a second," I interjected. "Do you realize how quickly you passed over a huge revelation about you and Phillip?"

"I know," she admitted, adding, "Do you think it's all right for me to see him?"

"I'm not here to pass any moral judgment. I know that dementia commonly has a huge impact on relationships and might lead to any number of unexpected situations."

As her friend and I listened, Claire explained that she and Robert had both known Phillip as a friend for some time. "He was there to help me on several occasions when handling Robert was difficult. One thing had led to another and the next thing we knew, we fell in love. Phillip is divorced. I even know his ex-wife. It's a pretty complicated set of circumstances. I guess that's why I overreacted about returning Robert to the adult family home. In my mind, it wasn't doing a good enough job—to me that was the cause of his depression—and I wanted him to receive the best care possible. "

She went on to explain that she had tried to talk about it with other friends, some who had known Phillip. In response, she received a full spectrum of reactions.

"Some friends seemed to completely understand, while others expressed mixed emotions. Two close friends are furious with me for what they perceived as my abandonment of my partner. This was upsetting, but the worst was yet to come.

"After receiving a halfhearted thumbs-up from my brother, I finally got up the nerve to discuss my feelings with my mother and father. They are in their 80s and strongly Catholic. They love Robert like a son. Not surprisingly, their reaction was severe. My father, with whom I could always talk, was very disappointed in me but was able to understand my side of it. He said that he supported my decision not to marry Robert when we decided to live together. Because we didn't make that commitment, from his perspective I was not bound to him. But my mother, who also was appalled when we decided not to marry, felt the other way. Her point of view was that, over so many years, we were together, and I had no business abandoning him. She is so upset she won't talk to me.

"I realized that I needed deeper support and turned to the Church. After I miscarried a baby in my early 40s, Father McCallister was so understanding and empathetic, even though Robert and I weren't married, that I sought him out again. I knew that he lost his mother to dementia, so I believed that he would be empathetic. And I was right. Yes, he reminded me that what I was doing was against the Church's doctrine, but while he could not condone my actions, he understood and accepted my decision. I will be forever grateful to him."

Such situations remind me continuously of why I like my work so much. Of course I don't I like to see people suffer over tough and life-changing decisions. But one of the reasons I went into psychiatry was because of the amazing diversity we all have, not just in terms of psychology, but in our beliefs—in the ethical, cultural, and moral values that color our life choices. Nowhere else have I seen this to be more prominent than in cases involving dementia.

For a healthy partner, making decisions on how to proceed in a relationship with a partner who has dementia can be daunting. Emotional needs may contrast with previous commitments; reality may contrast with hopes and dreams. And the situation is always changing because of the progressive nature of the disease. It is important not to make decisions in isolation. I encourage healthy partners to speak with those they trust about their feelings. Friends and family are one option but they may have a biased view or be too close to the situation to be objective. A dementia support group may be the best option, providing a variety of perspectives and support.

## OUTSIDE THE GROUP

There are people who make their decisions public. One such person is Barry Petersen, the CBS correspondent, whose wife, Jan Chorlton, also a well-known journalist, developed early onset Alzheimer's at the age of 55. In 2010 on CBS's *Sunday Morning*, Barry filed a report recounting the story of Jan's illness and why he decided to move her in to an assisted living facility. He also discussed why, on the advice of her mother, he had formed a relationship with another woman, a widow named Mary. Barry also documented what happened in a book, cowritten with Katie Couric, titled *Jan's Story: Love Lost to the Long Goodbye of Alzheimer's*.

Barry and Mary visit Jan together and share the decisions in directing her care—they consider themselves a sort of threesome family. Barry has told Mary that he would never divorce Jan.

I had the pleasure of being cospeaker with Barry at the 2011 Washington State Alzheimer's caregivers' conference sponsored by the University of Washington. There he expanded on the nature of his relationship with Jan, and what it was like to watch his life companion, as well as their romance, dwindle. He could no longer deal with Jan's aggression and other behaviors on his own. He says of those he knows who personally criticize him for his choices that, "it's okay, because they miss Jan."

There are people who undoubtedly feel that in Jan's case her husband must not have felt much for her, based upon his choices. However, Barry would tell you that this view couldn't be further from the truth.

From my perspective, I could understand. Jan had lost so much, and though Barry still loved and supported her, she couldn't even recognize him. Was it right that he should suffer the loss of so much without the love and support of someone else? Weren't his emotional needs important, too?

These are obviously difficult and private decisions that are not taken lightly. Yet as we now move into a world with more and more similar situations, woven into a tapestry of advanced technology and communication, it will be interesting to see what impact dementia and sex might have on a variety of aspects of our lives.

CHAPTER FIVE

# Sexuality in Long-Term Care

For many dementia patients, long-term care is a necessity. The reasons range from the patient needing more care than a partner can continue to provide, to partner burnout, to not being able to afford to pay for care at home. The long-term care facility, because of its close quarters, is often the scene of problematic sexual behavior. How the behavior is handled by facilities, staff, and families is yet another aspect of dealing with dementia.

## THE HEALTH CARE CHALLENGE

We are now, in 2013, at the beginning of the aging baby boomer phenomenon. This group, born between 1946 and 1965, started turning 65 in 2011. The resulting surge in the elderly population is expected to last about 18 years.

Add to that the fact that we are all living longer due to such factors as improved medical care and safety awareness, and the reality is that there are a lot of older people in America—and the numbers will keep growing. A variety of social, psychological, and medical concerns will affect each of us as we age. Personal losses, medical challenges, and difficulties in just "carrying on" are ahead for all who get older.

From the time we become sexually mature and begin the separation process from our parents, most of us never give a second thought to such basic tasks as brushing our teeth, going to appointments, feeding ourselves, or even hobbling around after an injury. Even with a pair of crutches and a cast, our habits, our peculiarities—even our sexuality—are always a part of us, ready to go, as privately and as actively as we desire.

But what if there came a point when things were no longer so private? With age comes the likelihood that we might need some help with those tasks so taken for granted. It may only be a sporadic need, especially early on, maybe as a result of a fall or a fracture. Yet, over time, the likelihood increases that help will be needed for the longer term.

Two-thirds of people 65 or older will require, in their lifetime, some long-term care at home—through adult day health care, like a visiting nurse service—or care in either an assisted living facility (ALF) or in a nursing home. If you buy long-term care insurance at age 60, there is a 50-50 chance you will use it. And though most long-term care in the United States is at home, over 40 percent of affected people will need a stay in a nursing home for some period of time—women average nearly four years, men two.

If you add up these numbers it's easy to see that the sum is a staggering amount of people, most of whom still have some habits, some peculiarities, and some sex life—and maybe a lot of the latter. Then factor in the possibility of dementia. What happens then?

## THE LANDSCAPE OF LONG-TERM CARE

Let's begin at home. For many, staying at home is preferred for a deep and fundamental reason: home is where people want to stay because no one, whether or not they are with a loved one, wants to lose his or her privacy.

Yet the equation involving home sometimes changes over time. Medical problems mount, especially when dementia enters the picture. The cost of home care can become astronomical, and even without that, caregiving burdens on the part of the spouse or partner or family will skyrocket. Plus, over time, the fight to preserve the privacy and independence of the caregivers themselves often is the crisis that changes everything.

When care is needed outside the home, the options, in general, are straightforward: ALFs, skilled nursing facilities (SNFs), and adult family homes (AFHs). The manner in which each of these options deals with private matters, including sex, can vary greatly.

Unless they have staff trained and dedicated specifically to provide dementia care, most facilities have little awareness or understanding of their patients' sexual needs beyond the demands of vague governmental regulations. For example, a confused man making repeated flirtatious remarks to the staff or other patients is taken back to his room and left alone, only to repeat the behavior over and over again. Eventually a staff member may make a request to the primary doctor for a drug to calm him down. Meanwhile, it's all too likely that no one took the time or recognized the possibility that he may have any number of needs generating the flirtation. Those could include a loss, loneliness, or genuine sexual needs that possibly could be expressed in a more private and appropriate way with some guidance from properly trained staff.

## ASSISTED LIVING FACILITIES

ALFs tend to be the higher-end facilities. They usually do not accept Medicaid, relying instead on payment from private funds or from long-term care insurance. They are often appealing settings, configured and detailed with a concern for those with confusion. Dementia care is often their strength, as they do not carry the nursing staff load of the SNFs, which usually deal with a variety of acute medical issues. The patients (or couples) may have their own private room. If a nurse, who has a key, wants to enter, he or she knocks on the door first. Understandably, for caregiving and health reasons, the expected level of privacy is greatly diminished, but that doesn't negate the fact that those in their room still may feel intruded upon.

There is a challenge for staff as well, since they might be entering a room where virtually anything could be happening. At a minimum, they are trained to respect privacy—that is, to properly announce themselves. While most staff is well received, they must sometimes field the anger and resentment that can occur when they are interrupting private moments that might include masturbation, sex with a spouse, or sex with another resident. Staff must do a very quick inventory of all these situations and determine safety, appropriateness, and any element of neglect or abuse, while at the same time fielding anger and frustration over their intrusion. The staff is not checking up on residents. What they are doing is giving prescribed medical care, such as timing their arriving to when it is time to administer a shot of insulin already drawn in the syringe. And if the nurse has 20 other patients to medicate, at some point sexual activity will be interrupted.

What happens if a female nurse enters the room where Hal is masturbating, and he keeps on masturbating—all the while smiling? What if he invites her to join in? What if Hal's wife is present? Now, the nurse's professional boundaries have been violated and it is she that feels compromised and vulnerable. Hopefully, she is trained and experienced enough to manage the situation professionally. That wasn't exactly the case with Lucy and Bruce.

Few spouses or partners expect or know how to handle sexual relationships that form in long-term care facilities. Yet the physical attraction between two people afflicted with dementia is a very common event. It doesn't really require a whole lot of maturity or professionalism to experience the common initial reaction that medical personnel feel, which is to separate the "cute" little couple. Unfortunately, things can become more complicated than that.

A few years back, I was called on my cell phone by a frantic executive director at a highly respected ALF that specialized in all levels of dementia care. It seemed that there was an extremely serious situation. The state surveyor was requiring that an outside consultant be called in immediately to provide training to all staff on the "identification, prevention, and reporting of abuse and neglect." I understood immediately why the director was so upset. Knowing something about long-term care, I was familiar with the use of the words neglect and abuse. The reputations of many dementia care facilities have been destroyed by those words. I agreed to the job. As part of the investigation, I was to review the policies and procedures and offer direction and training for the staff on the state laws and regulations.

The next morning I found myself on-site, behind closed doors and in front of the executive director and her boss. Corporate had been called in. It was bad. They were in "stop placement." This meant that the facility was not allowed to accept any new patients until the situation was resolved.

What had happened? The incident that triggered the reaction went back about a year or so. Lucy and Bruce were two residents at this ALF. They were admitted by their families because of the facility's reputation for providing the best dementia care around. And with that, presumably, would come the highest possible quality of life, including an immersion into whatever activities were deemed appropriate and that the residents could tolerate. The latter is a common expectation of dementia care facilities.

Lucy's spouse of 64 years had passed away about a year before, which, in part, led to her mental deterioration and the need for more care. As her children described it, their parents had enjoyed a committed and fulfilling relationship. Bruce was still married to Gloria, his wife of 60 plus years. This relationship was also described as loving and solid. At this point in time, however, Gloria was no longer able to care for Bruce at home. Reluctantly, she agreed to a trial of assisted living for him. Finding that he was thriving, she felt assuaged of her guilt and relieved to be able to move on with her friends and social activities.

Despite their relative proximity, Lucy's family was scarce when it came to visitation, although they responded quickly to any needs requested over the phone by staff, such as clothing or other supplies. On the other hand, some member of Bruce's family was there to visit almost daily. Because of that, Bruce's family was much more familiar with the development of a relationship between Bruce and Lucy.

What started between them as talk at the breakfast table progressed over a few months to hand holding. Finally, one day Gloria found her husband and Lucy lying together, clothed and calm, on his bed. The startled staff was more concerned about what Gloria's reaction might be, but fortunately she was collected. She even managed to maintain her composure when Bruce asked her who she was and explained that he was just relaxing on the bed with his wife.

Gloria later told me that she knew at that moment that he had moved on. She made it known to the staff that the relationship between the couple was acceptable to her, including whatever romantic interludes were to occur, as long as neither one was harmed. "You reach a point," she said, "after so many years together, where your partner being happy is the most important thing. There is no such thing as betrayal when it comes to this disease; in fact, it is the disease that is the betrayal."

Within a month, the evening staff informed her that Bruce and Lucy had been allowed to have sex.

Lucy, on the other hand, appeared to be the more passive partner. According to the staff, Lucy, who I never met, didn't seem to know who Bruce was and just went along with whatever he wanted to do. Uncomfortable with this, one of the evening nursing assistants called her family. The reaction was one of utter shock. They called the sheriff, who arrived that evening to investigate a case of rape as reported by the family. Lucy was taken to a local hospital and given a full rape evaluation, including a pelvic examination that required tranquilization after she became agitated. Discharged from the facility by her family and taken elsewhere, Lucy was never to be seen again by Bruce or anyone else there. I was certain a huge lawsuit was looming.

One could see Lucy's family's position on the events, but the facility was blatantly at fault for not informing them. After some review of the regulations, we accomplished the required staff education quickly. The state had also determined that the policies and procedures of the facility were inadequate in dealing with the situation, in particular with regard to abuse. At this point, the facility fired back that a primary mission of any dementia care facility was to provide for as many opportunities as possible to allow for the highest possible quality of life. The surveyors were reminded that this language in the federal regulations appeared in the state regulations as well.

This rebuttal changed the focus of the complaint. Now the facility was accused of not following the proper chain of command, which would have informed both families formally and given them proper opportunity to make the health care decision for their loved ones. The facility received what amounted to a slap on the wrist: it lost money due to a stop placement period. After the staff was retrained, the stop placement was lifted.

So what can be done in these kinds of delicate situations? How can families, staff, and patients cope? An open conversation involving family, staff, and, to the degree they can, the patients involved, along with a sound policy consistent with the state and federal regulations, is necessary to deal effectively with these complex and sensitive matters. There is often no right answer but rather a collection of views that, when aligned and consistent with the regulations, will lead to a solution.

Meeting with the staff, who were familiar with the tendency of patients to become involved with each other, we talked about options.

"Could Bruce's delusion about Lucy being his wife be treated with medication?" was the question one aide raised.

"What about Lucy's passivity?" a nurse asked. "Didn't that create a predatory situation, given her inability to make a choice?"

"I don't agree with that," another nurse chimed in. "Lucy, despite her passiveness, never seemed distressed. It didn't seem like she was enduring any neglect or abuse."

The longer the session went on the clearer it became that the thing for me to do was just to listen and allow them to express their opinions and emotions. This facility had clearly not offered such a venue for them. Although not directly admonished for this by the state, this seemed to me to be as critical an omission on the part of the facility as any of the other oversights.

One thing that stands out for me in cases like these is the ethical disparity of views from the staff: some feel that sex between patients is okay, and others are totally against it. These differences, in my mind, are healthy, and I will always work toward a solution, but only when both sides are allowed to express themselves openly. Sometimes staff members decide to leave or families may go elsewhere for care. But at least the differences are ironed out and dealt with in a controlled fashion, so as little harm as possible is done to the residents.

As for Gloria, she helped Bruce grieve his loss of Lucy by providing opportunities to talk about her. Still, it wasn't long before he forgot her. Ironically, he did remember, from time to time, who Gloria was. She was glad that, in his mind, she and Bruce were together romantically one last time before his memory faded even more. "Being with Lucy made him feel good," she said. "How could I deny him that? In a strange way, I felt his connection to me through Lucy, and for that I am grateful."

When appropriately managed, residents should have as much access to the full spectrum of human existence as possible, including sexual activity, if that is their desire. In my experience, this is healthy from a mental health standpoint because it limits psychiatric symptoms and the need for medications. Additionally, to do otherwise is a form of restraint. This freedom may also be representative of other thoughtful allowances that a particular facility has been able and willing to offer its residents. A good question to ask upon a visit, when considering placement of a family member, is "do you allow your patients to have sexual activity if the appropriate channels and considerations have been addressed?"

Another thoughtful allowance that might be visible, and should be a plus to a potential client in considering a facility, is the safe and monitored wandering of patients into spaces that a family might initially find strange. These include the administrator's office or nurses' station. Such tolerance shows savvy and experience and that the consideration of the patient is paramount.

## SKILLED NURSING FACILITIES

In the world of long-term care, SNFs are also known as rehab. Practically synonymous with long-term care, these used to be called nursing homes. Ironically, most of them would like nothing more than to provide short-term care. They feature the highest level of nursing and are the most hospital-like of the long-term care types, thus making them perfect as a step-down facility from the hospital for people with medical issues, such as hip fracture surgery or pneumonia, who are not able to return home straight away. Medicare Part A happens to fit into this model of care, covering most of the cost for up to 90 days.

Unfortunately "Med A," as it is referred to, will not cover any dementia care, as this will always be a longer term medical problem. Since most of those with money or long-term care insurance will look at ALF memory care first, due to their reputations and attractive appearances, the SNFs are often left with the relatively poorer Medicaid patients when it comes to dementia care. And with Medicaid comes a lower reimbursement. This plays a role in the wide spectrum of appearance in the SNFs. Some are majestic, while others are quite plain and even ugly. Most are in-between.

SNFs are the most highly regulated of long-term care facilities and must operate at a certain level or they will be shut down. Yet what you see on the outside is often reflected on the inside when it comes to amenities and patient privacy. Most facilities have a general focus, perhaps with a rehab/Med A wing and a dementia wing, but commonly the patients wander. When they wander, it's not uncommon for dementia patients to expose themselves or masturbate publicly. This kind of public behavior is not acceptable in any long-term care setting, but all privacy is limited. The rooms of an SNF tend to be double beds with a cloth pull barrier between them, so roommate interactions can become tricky.

Jim was a 71-year-old man, married and living at home with his wife. Retirement was going great until he fell and broke his hip. Fortunately, the surgery went well and he was admitted to an SNF for rehabilitation. This particular facility was a general one, with about a 50-50 mix of rehab and long-term care. The facility itself was old but was known for its staff of excellent physical therapists, and it was close to home, so Jim's wife could visit easily. At this time, the facility was full.

Jim's roommate, Rob, was a 68-year-old man with a similar fracture who was also there for rehab. They were placed together intentionally due to a similarity in age and diagnosis. However, Rob had a known history of mild dementia as well.

Both wives visited each evening and would then leave, sometimes together. One night, Rob's wife brought in a small television, which Jim didn't quite understand. A TV implied that Rob was inclined to stay for a while, whereas Jim was focused on getting out of the facility ASAP.

After the wives left, the TV went on and stayed on, with the volume fairly high. Jim confronted Rob, who only became increasingly irritable. Then Jim noticed that Rob was talking to himself as 11:00 o'clock turned to midnight and even later. Unable to bear his own weight, he asked Rob one last time if he would lower the TV. "Shut the fuck up, asshole," was the response. Jim pushed the call light for 20 minutes with no response. Finally, he yelled for help, which resulted in Rob turning the TV volume higher. The busy aide finally arrived about the same time that Jim began to smell feces.

Rob, confused and disoriented, had soiled himself. The aide pulled the curtain and called for help to get him changed. Two more aides soon arrived, but the fireworks were only getting started. Rob needed a full change, including bed linen. For Jim, the commotion was upsetting and frustrating. All he wanted to do was get some sleep.

Once the aides had Rob's clothes off, his mood seemed to change. Things got quieter for a while, but then came a series of exchanges through the curtain that practically put Jim into a state of disbelief. Rob began to rant some of the most vile and provocative sexual comments and requests that Jim had ever heard.

What impressed Jim most was the professional and neutral way the aides handled it all. He realized that if such a situation had occurred anywhere else, for instance in a bar or in a store, Rob could have been seriously injured. Instead, he got a new pair of pajamas and bedding, the TV was turned off, the light turned down, and some sort of medication was administered. Within minutes, Rob was snoring.

The next morning Rob was placed in another room by the administrator and director of nursing, both of whom apologized to Jim and his wife. Jim stayed for another week and completed his rehab. He returned home with a new respect for the privacy of his life.

## ADULT FAMILY HOMES

AFHs are on the rise. The reasons are clear: The SNFs want to do rehab and most of the ALFs are too expensive. If you can't be at home, and neither an SNF nor an ALF works out, the other option is an AFH. Generally based upon Medicaid reimbursement, these long-term care facilities are actually private residences converted into a place to care for those with disabilities.

The quality of care at AFHs can vary greatly. Some, with a waiting list a mile long, may have an absolutely fantastic reputation for giving the best dementia care imaginable, while others are downright scary. I would say that most, despite the relatively limited regulatory requirements, do provide good care. They are small, usually housing up to eight residents. As one might imagine, they allow for a more intimate setting, and this usually means more privacy for dementia residents. This is not as important to the actual residents as it might be to staff and families who might want to keep people separated from each other's sexual behaviors.

Karen was a woman who attended a talk I gave on sexual behavior and dementia. She told a story that related another advantage of an AFH. She and her husband Edgar had always enjoyed their sex life and continued to do so well into his dementia. But other behaviors, as well as safety and caregiving issues, had forced her to make a decision about long-term care. Karen chose an AFH because it met her requirements for expenses, location, and quality of care.

Edgar settled in quickly, and the owner lived up to her reputation by giving him the TLC that Karen had expected. Additionally, due to the smaller venue, Karen and the owner were able to make a plan for the continuation of her sex life with her husband. Karen spent every Friday night at the home. It was a fulfilling experience for the couple, even though he barely remembered who she was. In the morning, they would share breakfast with the other residents. Edgar would always thank his wife for coming to share the meal with them, having already forgotten the night they had just spent together.

## EXPECTATIONS VERSUS RIGHTS

There is a great deal of disparity between the different types of long-term care with regard to both appearance and care. Staff, from administrators to nursing assistants, will have varying degrees of experience, talents, or moral perspectives. Even levels of dedication to the mission of caring for the elderly and disabled will be inconsistent between staff members. In long-term care, money or long-term care insurance will buy a pleasant environment—for instance, a nice ALF. On the other hand, Karen and Edgar did just fine on a Medicaid budget at an AFH. Jim, who stayed at an SNF, had some extra money that might have paid for a private room in his relatively short rehab situation. But many like him would have allowed Medicare Part A to handle it all, considering the limited budgets of retirement.

Beyond researching the facilities, the finances, and the geography, combined with just plain luck, there remains the clinical reality that medically sicker patients may require skilled nursing. It's also necessary to factor into the equation that sexual behaviors can severely limit the choices available. Those with sexual behaviors will get onto the long-term care radar quickly in a very close-knit industry and will not be considered for admittance at most facilities. Because facilities have an obligation to keep other patents safe, contend with family, and meet regulatory standards, they view patients with sexual behavioral issues as potentially dangerous. The path to standards has taken decades.

In addition to understanding the sexual freedoms in a facility, families should also be concerned about safety and protection from sexual predation. Sexual incidents are required reports in all long-term care facilities and should be on public record. In many states it is mandatory to have this information, along with recent surveys, readily available and visible at the facility. During a tour, an open conversation with the administrator on this subject is a must. A discussion regarding policies and procedures, staff training and views on safety, and abuse versus patient rights should be included.

The federal government first got involved with long-term care in 1935 with the advent of Social Security. Debate occurred through the 1950s, but the next big change with upgraded regulations occurred in 1965 with the advent of Medicaid and Medicare. More changes were debated through the 1970s, but the current regulations were instituted as part of The Nursing Home Reform Act of 1987, which was legislated to address neglect and abuse in facilities accepting Medicaid and Medicare (which most do). States are required to adopt the federal standards at a minimum and to regulate the non-Medicaid and Medicare facilities as well.

There are specific federal regulations with which facilities must comply if they want any Medicaid or Medicare funding. There is little mention about sexual behavior in the act, yet there are plenty of gray areas that might affect someone's sexuality, such as rights to expression, privacy, and protection. (See chapter 10 for suggestions on updating the regulations, especially in regard to addressing the need for more specific and detailed direction on sexual issues.)

The state regulations generally cover similar issues, and sometimes in more detail. All states tend to focus on two things: the right to the basic privileges of living—food, sleep, socialization, and so on—and the right to safety from harm and abuse. The latter is a particularly thorny problem.

## ELDER SEXUAL ABUSE

If there is an antithesis to the freedom to engage in appropriately monitored sexual activity in long-term care dementia patients, it is sexual abuse. While this can take different forms, from predatory behavior to episodic inappropriate comments or actions, abuse remains a core concern for long-term care facilities, as reports of abuse can shut a facility down. Families may be less aware that this is even a possibility.

Signs of abuse may range from physical trauma, such as vaginal bleeding, to observations of inappropriate behaviors—including feeling uncomfortable—to actual reports by patients. And it may be the case that a family member is the perpetrator. Regardless, families should report immediately any concerns they may have regarding abuse of any kind, including sexual.

Staff would be expected to be less surprised by such events, but nonetheless they are trained to identify inappropriate behavior, intervene when safety is a concern, and report the concern immediately.

Research by physicians, sociologists, psychologists, and other health care professions reports that sexual assault on the elderly is underreported and understudied. It has been estimated that 5 to 10 percent of all elderly suffer from some degree of abuse, and that 5 percent of those cases involve some sort of sexual assault. Most victims of elder sexual abuse are women, and most perpetrators are men. Sexual abuse in the elderly may occur in the home or in a facility, and may be perpetrated by partners, relatives, caretakers, or others in a facility.

The highest incidence of elder sexual abuse—70 percent of reported cases—occurs in nursing homes. A reason for this may be, in part, due to the high degree of scrutiny that SNFs are under, thus mandating them to report incidents. However, a common citation against nursing homes relative to abuse is the failure to report it. Perpetrators within SNFs appear to be a mix of staff and patients.

Particular vulnerabilities to sexual assault in the elderly include physical weakness and cognitive deficit or dementia. The nature of the assaults may range from forced witnessing of, and exposure to, physical assault. Elderly sexual assault commonly involves genital injury, as well as fracture and injury to other parts of the body.

Now and then I meet for coffee with Ann, a nurse at a local SNF where I consult. We go back and forth on a variety of issues concerning long-term care. One of her more memorable stories was about the day she walked, holding a cup of medication, toward a room of two ladies with dementia. As she approached the doorway from the corridor, she saw one lady standing by the sink with a smile on her face looking across the room. This humored Ann. "Carol," she asked, "what's so funny?" As Ann entered the room she was then able to see what Carol was smiling at. Her roommate, Margaret, was naked on her bed. Gerald, who also suffered with dementia, was on the bed, too. He was straddling Margaret and trying to pry her legs open, as she struggled against him, though she was still obviously confused and uncertain about what was happening.

"In retrospect," Ann told me, "I should have just calmly separated them—but it's not every day that you walk in on a rape!"

Instead, Ann screamed for help and rushed to the couple on the bed. The result was that both apparent victim and perpetrator became agitated, as though Ann was interrupting sex between an established couple. As far as Ann knew, they were far from that, yet Margaret began scratching wildly at Ann and Gerald punched the nurse in the face before others arrived.

Per protocol, the case was reviewed by the facility and the state. Gerald, a known sexual predator in the past, was not adequately monitored or supervised. Margaret, examined at a hospital, was found to be unharmed, yet the process of a rape examination was upsetting to her as she had little understanding of what was happening. Still, this was not her first such examination since she entered an SNF. Her medical records detailed a vaginal tear from presumed physical contact at another facility.

It occurred to her insightful family that, psychologically, the incidents might have been related to the physical abuse she endured in her 50-year marriage. Perhaps that pattern made her submissive to predators. It was determined that, at the very least, her confusion made her vulnerable. Consequently, she was monitored more carefully.

## IMPROVING CARE

It seems that long-term care, for all of its goodwill and strengths, by its nature presents an impingement upon privacy for guests. This, in turn, may have an impact upon sexuality or even make one vulnerable to the sexuality of others. Yet with dementia care in general, social stimulation is generally considered to be a therapeutic plus. However, facilities have an obligation to provide for the preservation of as much dignity as possible and at the same time protect patients from neglect and abuse. The failure to protect is the number one citation that facilities receive from monitoring agencies when it comes to patient abuse. Number two is the failure to adopt a policy on the subject, and number three is the failure to report abuse in the first place.

Interestingly, while most reported elder abuse happens in long-term care facilities, it may be the regulation of the SNFs, ALFs, and AFHs that help to bring it to our attention. (It makes one wonder how much abuse is happening in private home situations where most dementia patients live and, due to lack of regulations, may be under- reported.) Moreover, it is incumbent upon facilities not only to protect residents, maintain an abuse policy, and report abuse, but also to be aware of each person's sexuality, beginning when the individual arrives at the front door. Specific staff training should encourage an openness to discuss elder sexuality: many elderly still masturbate or might seek a sexual partner. It might even be that what seems sexual or romantic to us might be more of a need to touch or even "cuddle" to someone who is confused. Still, staff should be trained on the facility operations manual and policies when it comes to sexual issues to help them recognize what is, and is not, acceptable behavior. And they must be aware of safety, such as the emergency procedure for getting help in a situation such as Ann's. They must learn what lines not to cross physically and emotionally. Staff must also learn to be cautious with rooming decisions and keep an eye on potential or identified sexual perpetrators. Finally, the staff in long-term care more often than not is mostly female. They must learn how to protect themselves from a potential assault as well.

Such awareness will lead to more openness about elder sexuality. This, in turn, will lead to greater opportunity to properly adjust the environment for each patient as much as possible and to report potential predation, including that of fellow staff members. The result will provide the greatest and fullest possible life experience while at the facility, with the greatest degree of protection for patients and staff alike.

As you read in part one, dealing with sexuality and dementia requires the understanding of many things, including what happens to the brain and the impact of sexuality and dementia on society, in relationships, and in long-term care. In the next part of the book, the chapters will focus on age-related and other dementias, the sexual effects of delirium, drugs, and other substances, and how symptoms are treated. The final chapter will offer suggestions for changing the way dementia is treated and regarded.

With this knowledge in hand, you will be able to recognize the types of dementia and the spectrum of sexual troubles, and you will become familiar with the available treatments. Doing so will make you better prepared to cope with your particular situation.

PART TWO

# Understanding What You Are Facing

CHAPTER SIX

# Age-Related Dementia

A dementia care home where I consult is a little different than most I visit because instead of being in the suburbs, it's located in a downtown/urban area. Buses and cars continuously cruise by, interrupted by the occasional honking fire truck, and the sidewalks are crowded with people. Inside the dementia care home, however, it's just like any other such facility. Nursing staff intermingles with the men and women playing cards, taking their medication, resting, or just wandering about. Elevator music plays in the background.

One of the challenges of all such facilities—the care for many people with dementia—is the safety and security of the patients. On occasion, someone will maneuver past whatever protection is in place and make it out of the facility, alone and free to do as he or she pleases.

Once while I was there, this scenario happened. The police were called and a search party was sent out. But I wondered: If people didn't know what the patient looked like, or exactly what he was wearing, how could they identify the missing person walking down a city street? What does a dementia patient look like out in public?

If you guessed "older" you would, of course, be right. Still, no particular physical characteristics are dementia indicators. Neither sex nor race is a factor, any more than skin conditions or hair color.

What about gait, the way someone walks? Stroke dementia can be associated with a one-sided paralysis (hemiparesis), but such patients would be in a wheelchair and not likely to get far. Besides, most stroke patients with a one-sided paralysis don't have dementia. While the motor area of the brain is affected by the stroke, there may not be a culmination of damage from smaller or even microscopic strokes in corresponding cognitive areas yet.

Parkinson's patients will eventually walk with a shuffling gait. Yet again, most Parkinson's patients don't have dementia—they will, however, develop it if they live long enough. Generally, a patient who wanders away onto the streets is likely to walk well, not shuffle, since the person must be physically intact enough to accomplish such a task.

The fact is that dementia patients, especially those in the majority with Alzheimer's, exhibit no apparent physical impairments, especially in the early or middle stages of the disease. Later on, sufferers forget how to walk rather than not being able to for some physical reason. This is called an apraxia and can be used to diagnose a dementia like Alzheimer's.

So, our missing dementia patient is likely older but not necessarily "real old," that is, in his 90s when confusion is seen more as a part of aging rather than a disease.

This person is probably walking and moving well with the same purposeful movements that got him out the door in the first place. What about the man who appears to be drunk, sitting on a stoop with a bottle of gin? He's not likely the missing person. Our patient has too many people to see and places to go. Short-term memory loss keeps him moving from one site to the next. He will be interested in lots of things, albeit briefly, so he won't be too different from anyone else browsing along the streets. Also, our runaway would not carry any cash. Residents aren't given money at the facility so that if they do wander away, they won't get far.

Behaviorally, he might seem perfectly normal. Much overt expression of psychosis or agitation is often linked to a lack of stimulation or confinement. This newfound freedom is a time for wandering and exploring and not being upset.

The attire of our patient is also normal. He likely looks just like anyone else; maybe some egg fell or coffee dripped on his shirt. Our patient might be talking to himself, but in a soft and private way, and not with the loud and boisterous rant of the schizophrenic whose clothes, like that of the alcoholic, are often worn and dirty, indicators of time on the streets. You never will see much wear and tear in a dementia patient as he lacks survival skills and will soon need aid. Like anyone with a Bluetooth device, it appears that he is talking to someone who isn't there. At the same time, he is observing what is going on around him.

Lacking inhibition, eventually our dementia patient will engage in a conversation with someone, and this will be how he will be discovered. He might ask for directions to a store in another city during a period of time long ago, or he might even flirt. If the conversation goes on for long, he will raise concerns and give himself away. Without short-term memory, the loss of which is the hallmark of most dementia, he will seem odd and unable to make sense. Being older and fragile, yet well-tended in terms of his dress and hygiene, will stand out as markers of his condition.

However, there are other indicators of age-related dementias.

***Symptoms from the Ground Up***

When I taught students at Columbia University Medical School how to do a quick physical examination in the Psychiatric Emergency Department, there was always surprise and amusement when I suggested that we start with the feet.

Here's why. Clipped nails, toenail polish, and clean feet with little callus are not generally seen in a chronic schizophrenic or an alcoholic living on the streets for long periods. Their hygiene, as opposed to those in dementia care facilities, generally ranges from poor to nonexistent.

## IDENTIFYING DEMENTIA

It's very common for dementia in older people to be bundled under the umbrella of Alzheimer's. And while all Alzheimer's disease is dementia, not all dementias are Alzheimer's. There are very particular markers of each of the four main causes of age-related dementia.

Alzheimer's, cerebrovascular disease (strokes), Lewy body disease, and Parkinson's disease are responsible for 90 percent of the dementia cases in the United States. At present, there is no cure for any of them, and each condition is ultimately fatal in that the patient will die earlier because of this illness. However, there is great variability here. While those with early onset Alzheimer's or Lewy body dementia might not live five years, others with Parkinson's disease or vascular dementia might live 15 or 20 years or, although rarely, more.

It has been reported that there is approximately a 5 percent prevalence in the combined 70- to 80-year-old group for dementia of all types, about 25 percent for the 80- to 90-year-olds and 40 percent for 90 and above. Other studies done in Europe showed similar numbers.

Dementia and old age are linked for good reason. The most common types of the disease in the United States (and in most industrialized places in the world) list old age as the primary risk factor. However, old age involves quite a range. While someone in a memory care facility is likely to be 70, 80, or more years old, there are others who are 50 or 60.

There are four major causes of dementia:

- Alzheimer's disease, the most common form of dementia in the United States, is responsible for about 60 percent of cases there and about 50 percent worldwide.
- Vascular, or stroke-related dementia, the second most common form, accounts for 20 percent of cases.
- Parkinson's disease and Lewy body disease together account for 15 to 20 percent of cases, with an estimate of 70 percent of those cases caused by Parkinson's disease.

It is also important to note that there is a great deal of overlap; many patients with Alzheimer's dementia have some degree of stroke disease. Additionally, there are forms of Alzheimer's with features of Lewy body and Parkinson's diseases.

## ALZHEIMER'S DISEASE

The onset of this cruel disease is slow and insidious, making for the perfect opportunity for denial, which is almost always the case on the part of the patient and is common on the part of the family as well. Sometimes a partner can't see the changes taking place over time. That was the situation for Tom and Molly.

When Tom and Molly were nearly 70 years old, they decided it was time for a change. The kids were gone, the bills were minimal, they were well off financially, and they were seemingly healthy. It was time for a long vacation.

Molly had always wanted to see Scandinavia, where her parents were from. Tom was hesitantly agreeable, so given that there was plenty of family to stay with abroad, Molly planned a three-month excursion. This prompted their youngest daughter, Debbie, to make a move of her own. Since she was able to telecommute to her job, she decided to live in her parents' house while they were away.

Debbie arrived a week before the trip to spend time with her parents whom she had not seen in nearly two years. I remember her telling me how astounded she was after talking with her dad for the first few minutes after she arrived.

"It was as if, emotionally, he was made of plastic. It wasn't really a physical thing as much as his demeanor. He was apathetic and unable to go very far in a conversation. I asked if he was depressed. He said no, that he felt well. He seemed to eat and sleep okay."

She went on. "Later that night I had a chance to talk with mom. She thought he was fine, but I knew something was wrong, and I wasn't going to let it go. It turned out that mom had taken over the checkbook and driving, two things that dad always did. She told me that they no longer went out regularly with a good friend—a relationship that had been ongoing for years before it was stopped.

"On the other hand, mom said they were doing well together, that they were closer than ever. They even put their wedding rings back on after years of keeping them in a drawer. Mom said that dad was even chasing after her around the house. At first I thought he was getting violent with her until she smiled about it. Then I understood: they were actually having sex.

"But dad, who loved to tinker with his two old cars in the garage hadn't been out there in over a year. I asked mom if she had mentioned any of this to the doctor. She said the doctor only asked how things were going, and they said fine—which they were, according to her."

A progressive decline: This is classic Alzheimer's disease, marked by cognitive decline with significant dysfunction in an aging but otherwise healthy individual. The gradual onset had allowed Molly to step in and take over without noticing a thing missing, but Debbie had gotten a sudden two-year dose of change. The snapshot she saw was alarming.

Debbie got her dad to the doctor right away. It was clear on examination that his short-term memory abilities were severely impaired. Debbie was understandably peeved that the doctor hadn't picked up on this earlier. (The doctor's oversight was, sadly, not unusual. Many primary care doctors don't routinely screen for memory loss, attributing it to normal aging.)

As mentioned in chapter 3, a common feature of Alzheimer's appears to be the secretion of a toxic plaque called beta amyloid, which, in turn, generates an inflammatory response around the neurons, killing them. The hippocampus, which is crucial to forming new memories, is one particular area affected by Alzheimer's. As there is no blood test for Alzheimer's, identifying memory loss alone should bring one well down the path toward the diagnosis. The rest is a matter of ruling out other problems, such as different forms of dementia or brain concerns, with a computerized axial tomography (CT) or magnetic resonance imaging (MRI) scan, along with tests for low thyroid and low vitamin B12 levels, and addressing possible medical confusion or delirium. Also, depression or other mental illness should be ruled out.

Debbie later asked me what her father's condition meant for her in terms of genetic risk. I told her that only 10 percent of cases are "familial" and highly genetic, where many members of each generation get the disease. Like Parkinson's disease, most cases are considered sporadic. The role of genetics in the other 90 percent of cases is unclear, although the APoE4 gene is believed to play a role.

There are four types of APoE genes: 1, 2, 3, and 4. APoE4 has been linked to cardiovascular disease, poorer outcomes after brain trauma, and an increased risk of Alzheimer's disease. Those with two APoE4 genes (one from each parent) face a 10 to 30 percent increase in the risk of developing Alzheimer's disease.

One question in the genetics of Alzheimer's discussion is whether or not this disease may, more often than not, occur in its pure form. That is, the typical degenerative changes of Alzheimer's are found without evidence of other causes of dementia like strokes or Lewy bodies.

It is known from studies, for example, that there is a significant amount of stroke disease in those previously diagnosed with Alzheimer's disease.

One of the trends in research over the past decade has been a noticeable relationship between some risk factors for stroke and Alzheimer's such as hypertension, high cholesterol, and diabetes. By inference then, one might get the idea—correctly in my view—that the genetic risks of hypertension, diabetes, and high cholesterol apply to the overall risk of being diagnosed with Alzheimer's.

Beyond the genetic risks, it has become clear that lifestyle choices are a major factor in brain health as well, particularly as it relates to strokes. This seems to have two important elements. First, making an effort to work with a health care provider to manage existing health problems like hypertension, diabetes, and high cholesterol clearly results in a lessening of the impact they might have on the body. Secondly, such problems can be limited, or even prevented from developing, with a personal commitment to better health through nutrition, exercise, and proper stress management.

### *Ten Questions Your Doctor Should Ask*

Memory loss causing noticeable degrees of social dysfunction in a 70-year-old is not normal. A routine social history, such as changes of duties between the partners or social anxieties, should be performed in all elderly patients, along with routine memory screening. This should be a standard form that a spouse, partner, or family member should fill out. (The patient will never give an accurate report.)

Your doctor should ask you the following about the person with memory loss:

1. Have there been new problems with memory?
2. Have there been changes in mood?
3. Have there been changes in thinking, such as confusion?
4. Have there been changes in the relationship?
5. Is the spouse taking over duties previously done by the partner?
6. Is there a new social anxiety?
7. Is there nighttime wandering?
8. Have there been any trips or living situation changes and how was that tolerated?
9. Have there been hallucinations?
10. Have there been mistakes in identity of family or friends?

Additionally, there should be some objective standardized cognitive testing done in any suspicious case and possibly as a screen for anyone 65 or older. A commonly used example is the Folstein Mini Mental Status Examination (MMSE). This is an easy-to-use screen given to the patient that measures memory, awareness, and cognitive ability on a scale of 0 to 30.

## STROKE-RELATED DEMENTIA

A stroke is an area of the brain with a lack of blood supply that leads to cell death. This may occur as the result of a thrombus (a body of clotted blood), or an embolus (a piece of an atherosclerotic fatty plaque breaking off the wall of an artery that becomes lodged, creating a blockage). Another cause of stroke is hemorrhage. This may be traumatic or the result of a malformation. However, it is commonly the result of uncontrolled high blood pressure.

With age comes years of exposure to the medical risks of stroke. These include smoking, high-fat foods, stress, and genetic predisposition to the deposition of fat on the lining of the arteries. The plaques may break off but also there may be blood clots that travel. Atrial fibrillation (AF), a quivering of the upper part of the heart that leads to irregular intracardiac blood flow, is a common cause of blood clots. This is why all patients with AF are on blood thinners. Another cause of stroke is the direct effect of seriously high blood pressure that can cause blood vessels in the brain to burst on a microscopic or grand scale. When that happens, brain cells die. Strokes may be massive, involving a large area of the brain, or microscopic, accumulating a dangerous mass over time. In either case, brain tissue dies and clinical symptoms eventually begin to emerge.

But, unlike other dementias, the character of stroke dementia depends more on where the strokes occur.

A sudden stroke in one area might cause hypersexual behavior overnight in a relatively unconfused person. On the other hand, millions of microscopic-level strokes could wipe away someone's memory over the course of years. As a rule, stroke dementia tends to take a more step-like progression than Alzheimer's. The diagnosis is made by clinical examination—that is, strokes seen on radiographic studies—and ruling out other causes such as delirium or either Alzheimer's or Parkinson's.

That was the case with Bernard, a robust 67-year-old attorney whose African American heritage contributed to both high blood pressure and diabetes from an early age. By the time he was in his 50s, he suffered with some loss of both kidney and eye function due to microscopic stroke disease.

But for years prior to that he was not able to engage in usual sexual activity with his wife due to erectile dysfunction from microvascular stroke disease in the penis. Unfortunately, due to his eye disease, he was not considered a candidate for medication to help his erectile dysfunction. Yet, with all his conditions, he was only marginally compliant with his medication for his blood pressure, diet, or exercise. His doctor warned him that a big stroke was coming—and it did.

One night while in bed, Bernard seemed confused to his wife Tanya. His speech was garbled, and he didn't make sense. She noticed that the right side of his face and body were drooping and called 911. Rushed to the ER, Bernard arrived in time to receive treatment that saved some of the movement on his side. But he was left with an expressive aphasia, which is the inability to get the correct words out. He also experienced a pseudobulbar affect, the mood disorder characterized by involuntary and inappropriate laughing or crying commonly seen in stroke patients.

The unstable mood mixed with the speech impediment made for a nearly impossible situation, especially for an attorney who was used to speaking in court. Bernard was extremely frustrated, as was his wife. She was unable to care for him at home.

"What a disaster," Tanya told me. "I've never seen anything like this. Imagine a proud man unable to stop crying—even when he's not sad—and unable to get a damn word out edgewise. He went through so many rehabs and therapists over the past year … all that just took him over the edge."

When I looked at the MRI of Bernard's brain I could understand why Bernard and Tanya were struggling. His brain looked like the moon, cratered with strokes of all sizes. It was hard to imagine he wasn't significantly impaired cognitively. Of course he couldn't cope with all the treatments and changes in his life—the nursing rehab facilities, the loss of independence, the separation from Tanya. Bernard remained on treatment, another six months but still suffered some new stroke activity, with each event taking a little more of him away. He died about a year later of kidney failure while living at a nursing home.

***Exercise and Dementia***

A recently completed study demonstrated that improved physical fitness could reduce the risk for dementia in general. This included both patients with and without stroke disease. In this study, the fitness level of 20,000 people around 50 years old was measured. These people were then followed for 25 years.

*(continued)*

***Exercise and Dementia (continued)***

The study revealed that the risk of dementia was diminished by 36 percent in those with the higher starting fitness level over those with the lower. The author of the study felt that these results are consistent with the current U.S. physical activity guideline of 150 minutes of moderate exercise weekly.

Another study reported that a slowing in cognitive deterioration and disease-related brain changes was demonstrated when patients already suffering with dementia did 6 to 12 months of moderate regular exercise compared to sedentary patients.

## DEMENTIA WITH LEWY BODIES

Around the turn of the 20th century, the German neurologist Frederick Lewy discovered small protein bodies inside the cells of some patients with dementia. It would be decades before other scientists would gather enough information to realize that Lewy bodies played a huge role in the condition.

The cognitive hallmark of dementia with Lewy bodies (DLB) is fluctuations of attention or awareness throughout the day. Families commonly report long periods of the afflicted person seeming to float in and out of awareness.

Next, visual hallucinations may occur. It is important to note that outside of delirium, such hallucinations are not common symptoms, particularly in other forms of dementia.

The third hallmark of DLB is sensitivity to antipsychotic medications. It is the nature of Lewy body disease to destroy dopamine reserves in the brain. This is what is responsible for the symptoms of Parkinson's disease. It happens that antipsychotic medications also have a negative effect on this important neurotransmitter in creating a temporary blockade at the level of the synapse, the space between the brain cells. They can create a short-term Parkinsonism, a well-known side effect. Giving a dopamine-blocking drug to someone who is already depleted of it will exacerbate a problem with severe Parkinson's symptoms.

This is an important therapeutic point because patients with both DLB and Parkinson's disease dementia (PDD) often have psychotic symptoms—visual hallucinations and delusions—requiring treatment. Fortunately, Seroquel (quetiapine) is the one antipsychotic medication that is fairly well tolerated in such patients because it doesn't block dopamine as much as other antipsychotics do. For this reason, many patients with either DLB or PDD will be on this medication.

DLB is a much quicker and aggressive illness than Parkinson's because the Lewy bodies are found initially in the cortical thinking area of the brain and spread from there. It can also have features of Alzheimer's, such as the inability to form new memories. Most people diagnosed with DLB will not live 10 years past the point of diagnosis. Many are fighters who will not give up. Mathilda was such a person.

Stubborn and determined that others see her point of view, she never gave up anything without a verbal battle. She was also the rock her family leaned on. When she was diagnosed with DLB, George, her husband of 47 years, and their children were devastated. "It all came on so fast," George explained. "Last fall she was normal. We just thought she was depressed, but then the paranoia and confusion started culminating in a persisting idea that people were listening to her through the walls. A few years ago our house flooded during a storm, and we thought that the resulting mold might be the reason. But I was exposed just as much as she was, and I'm okay. She also started to experience some memory problems a couple of years ago, when she was 70, although she was healthy in every other way.

"Thank God we could bring her to this unit where she could check in and the medical team could figure this out. As awful as this is, Mathilda will make this the fight of her life."

George was right, but Mathilda was a terribly difficult patient to treat. She suffered with all kinds of side effects to the meds—when she took them: much of the time she was noncompliant. Additionally, she was confrontational and liked to try to belittle my staff and me.

Mathilda experienced regular visual hallucinations, as well as fluctuations of confusion common to DLB patients, and she was very sensitive to any antipsychotic drug with the exception of Seroquel. Fortunately, we were able to stabilize her, and she was able to return home with her husband and daughters who all lived nearby in a dairy farming community. As of this writing, she is still there.

## PARKINSON'S DISEASE DEMENTIA

While this is a disease of slow progression that can last 20 years, dementia usually starts 10 years after the onset, along with other symptoms such as visual hallucinations.

Treatment for Parkinson's disease, which generally begins in people in their 50s, 60s, and 70s, is initially generally effective and centered around dopamine replacement. Unfortunately, these treatments may eventually have their own debilitating side effects, especially after years of use. These include psychosis and irregular muscle movements called dyskinesias. Finding the right balance of medication can be tricky. Too little dopamine results in the classic Parkinson's symptoms of tremors and a shuffling gait. Too much dopamine is marked by dyskinesia, an irregular flailing movement.

In the case of Parkinson's disease, Lewy bodies are seen in the basal ganglia, a movement and mood area with lots of serotonin and dopamine. As the dopamine progressively deteriorates, the typical symptoms of the disease begin. Those symptoms include the mask-like disanimated face, slowed movements, slow tremor (usually greater on one side), and rigidity, all of which ultimately make life unbearable.

Some patients with Parkinson's disease live 20 to 30 years after diagnosis. However, as a group, there appears to be a shortened life span, similar to those who have had a heart attack. Developing PDD will further lower the long-term survivability of the illness. Studies vary, but it is estimated that some 50 to 80 percent of patients with Parkinson's disease will develop PDD within 10 years. That's what happened to a patient of mine.

Larry worked for the airlift wing in the Air Force, flying around the world to do his work. After years of raising their children on Air Force bases, Larry, and his wife Delia, decided to retire. Larry was diagnosed with Parkinson's several years into retirement. He tolerated his treatment well and remained relatively stable and active. At around age 65, about 10 years into the illness, he started to decline cognitively. His mood was more depressed, and his memory was failing. He began to see visions of his parents at the foot of his bed, which understandably distressed him. According to Delia, he would be "off one day and on the next. I'd hardly know he had dementia but then suddenly he seemed gone.

"And he's so depressed." She continued. "I've never seen a person so miserable. He traveled all around the world and *now* look at him. He can barely walk down the hall."

Eventually Larry required higher doses of Sinemet to keep him from freezing up with the Parkinson's symptoms, but the tradeoff was huge. He experienced the irregular movements of dyskinesia, along with paranoia. To offset the complications, doses of the Seroquel were increased. Then the movements got worse. Delia, along with Larry's medical team, were eventually forced to make a wrenching decision. Another tragedy of his condition was that Larry was too confused to express what he wanted.

"I know that the visions, along with the inability to stop moving, was killing Larry as much as the disease was. By this time Larry was ready to let go. We decided to take him off the meds, which left him unable to swallow or eat. Soon after the decision was made—the hardest thing we ever did—he developed pneumonia and died. As wrenching as his death was, I was relieved that his suffering was over."

### *Risk Factors for Developing Dementia*

Many people ask me if there are particular risk factors connected to developing dementia. There are some. The following list highlights factors, along with particular symptoms to watch for.

**Alzheimer's Disease**

A number of cases in a family history may indicate risk, but most pure cases of Alzheimer's disease are sporadic and can occur seemingly out of thin air. Limiting vascular risks, such as diabetes, high blood pressure, and high cholesterol, through diet, exercise, and proper medical care may have substantial impact, as many cases are mixed. Symptoms include:

- Progressive memory loss
- Social anxiety
- Inability to perform complex tasks

**Stroke-Related Dementia**

Those people with a history of hypertension, and/or diabetes, and/or high cholesterol are at heightened risks for stroke and the dementia that can result from it.

Symptoms include:

- Sudden or stepwise memory loss otherwise unexplained. In contrast to the "smooth" decline that occurs in Alzheimer's, little steps or "shelves" of decline, each represented by a new and sudden stroke, mark this type of dementia.

*(continued)*

***Risk Factors for Developing Dementia (continued)***

- Unstable moods
- Change in personality

**Lewy Body Dementia**

There is no obvious risk or genetic relationship for Lewy body dementia. Symptoms include:

- Parkinson's symptoms or sensitivity to antipsychotic medication
- Fluctuations of confusion
- Visual hallucinations

**Parkinson's Dementia**

About 15 percent of these cases are familial; there is a gene with a mutation that leads to the disease being passed down in the family. However, there is not one single gene mutation; different familial genes have been discovered. Most cases of Parkinson's, like Alzheimer's, occur spontaneously and are probably multifactorial, which would involve many genetic predispositions. This type of dementia will occur if the person with Parkinson's disease lives long enough for it to develop. Symptoms include:

- Memory loss
- Depression
- Visual hallucinations

## THE TREATMENTS

Efforts are underway to further understand these illnesses and what else can be done for sufferers, but for now much of the care is palliative management of the symptoms.

However, unlike 20 years ago, there are now several medications available to treat some of these conditions. Three of them, Aricept (donepezil), Exelon (rivastigmine), and Razadyne (galantamine) work by increasing the amount of acetylcholine in the brain. This is the neurotransmitter so integral to the formation of memory that is devastated in Alzheimer's and Lewy body dementia. The U.S. Food and Drug Administration (FDA) has approved Aricept and Razadyne for treating Alzheimer's dementia, while Exelon gained the additional approval for treatment of Parkinson's dementia.

A fourth medication, Namenda (memantine), helps to calm the toxic effects of overstimulation of the brain through the glutamate system. The drug is indicated only for Alzheimer's dementia (see chapter 8).

Due to the overall lack of therapeutic options, all of these medications are being used off-label for all types of dementia They have never been shown to change the disease state, nor has one been shown to work better than the other. They can buy time, however, which is something that families facing the hard realities of such illnesses can cherish.

CHAPTER SEVEN

# Other Dementias

While dementia is associated with people aged 50 and older, many men and women who are much younger are also affected. There are numerous reasons for these dementias. Some are linked to genetics, toxins, and head injuries, while others are the result of infections. Still others have no apparent cause. Some of these other dementias are aggressive, with death occurring quickly—in a year or so—while others linger, creating a long-term situation the patient and his or her family must deal with.

In this chapter, the focus will be on the dementias with a particular link with, or significance to, sexuality. They all tend to occur in younger patients but also differ in significant ways, such as in their prevalence, cause, or historical significance. (Alcohol dementia also occurs in the young. It will be discussed in detail in chapter 8: "The Sexual Effects of Delirium, Drugs, and Other Substances.")

Dementia in youth and middle age is not a new occurrence. However, one needs to remember that only 100 years ago the average age of death was much younger than it is today. Therefore, many of the classic dementias of older age didn't have the opportunity to occur as they do in the world full of older people we live in now. In the past, the dementia that existed was almost always in younger people. And while early onset forms of illnesses like Alzheimer's and Parkinson's probably did exist, in the past dementia was more likely related to trauma or infection.

From an infectious disease standpoint, there are two ravaging epidemics in particular, each closely linked to both sex and dementia. The first, neurosyphilis, is a bacterial illness that is important now more from a historical perspective than a current one. Aside from being transmitted sexually, it was associated with personality change, insanity, madness, and ultimately dementia. The second, HIV illness, has been a scourge of modern times. This is a viral illness, also transmitted sexually, with a path to dementia in many cases. Its described psychiatric scenarios seem somewhat tame compared with those of syphilis, undoubtedly in part due to modern treatments for psychosis and mood disorders, as well as more standard descriptive tools for psychiatric symptoms. Nonetheless, severe bouts of mania, depression, and psychosis have been described, leading, regrettably, to further irresponsible transmission of the disease.

## SYPHILIS: THE GREAT POX

To this day it remains unclear if the bacteria *Treponema pallidum*, which causes syphilis, was brought back to Europe by the Columbus expedition to the Americas or existed there already. Spread primarily through sexual contact with an open sore, syphilis was called the Great Pox, to distinguish it from smallpox, and was once considered one of the worst diseases known to man. It was feared as much as leprosy in Biblical times, and the Black Death—bubonic plague—in the 1400s in Europe. Early forms of the disease were particularly virulent, leading to severe body deformities as skin filled with pustules and bacteria-loaded tumors. Later, in the Renaissance, a less severe form allowed the numbers of afflicted to grow to numbers that rivaled those of the most infectious diseases. Its impact on the population was profound, killing as many as five million people throughout Europe from the time of Columbus through the Renaissance.

A variety of only marginally successful treatments prevailed, ranging from spiritualism, to purposeful infection with malaria from agents made of arsenic, to treatment by exposure to the metal mercury and all of its toxic effects. From this latter method came the saying, "a night in the arms of Venus leads to a lifetime with mercury."

No wonder that many afflicted opted to avoid treatment. Unfortunately, there is much more to this disease than a genital rash. The secondary phase is a body rash that might occur months after the initial infection. Finally, there is tertiary syphilis, which might severely affect the cardiovascular or nervous system. Syphilis is known as "the great imitator" because a disease-related skin rash, sore throat, or joint ache might be mistaken for the measles, strep throat, or influenza. To suffer such a disease progression would be to join the ranks of such famous men as Ivan the Terrible, Oscar Wilde, Adolf Hitler, and Al Capone. The latter reportedly went insane in prison due to the neurological consequences of the disease, and the other three are strongly suspected to have suffered from it.

A dramatic lessening of the prevalence of syphilis came in the 1900s with the discovery of antibiotics, and, in particular, penicillin in 1928. Up until then 10 to 15 percent of those in urban areas had the disease, with 25 percent of those cases going on to later stages. Considering that there are still millions of cases reported annually worldwide—90 percent of them in the Third World—this would be a serious neurological disease crisis if it weren't for the effectiveness of today's drugs. In the United States there was a resurgence of the disease in the '60s and '70s, presumably due to the advent of sexual liberation, and in the '80s and '90s due to a sex for crack cocaine exchange culture in inner cities. Since 2000 there has again been a rise of syphilis cases in the gay male population, along with those who are immunocompromised because of AIDS. Most recently, the baby boomers have been identified as a group with rising levels of sexually transmitted diseases, including syphilis. Fortunately, most such cases are recognized early and treated.

Rarely, some patients in the United States don't get treatment and the disease takes its course. In some cases, this might be due to resistant strains of the bacteria. In others, it might be due to lack of education or poor access to health care, with the disease going unrecognized because of its episodic and chameleon-like nature. It has been established that the spirochete bacteria causing syphilis will enter the central nervous system in some 25 percent of untreated cases. From there the disease might progress neurologically anywhere from 3 to 50 years after the initial infection. One of the known forms of neurosyphilis is called general paresis.

When paresis or "paralysis of the insane" is present, over time the spirochetes cause an inflammatory reaction in the cognitive areas of both the nerve cells and the blood vessels of the brain. The former causes cell death. The latter leads to microscopic strokes that do the same. Once identified, neurosyphilis is treated with aggressive intravenous penicillin therapy. Some of the cognitive deficits that might range from grandiose mood and personality changes to memory loss or confusion might turn around, to some degree, with treatment. However, the damage, such as enlarged ventricles or small stroke disease, often is already notable on a CT or MRI scan. Such changes are permanent, and so are the clinical findings. This is the dementia directly caused by syphilis. Years ago, I saw a case firsthand.

Gabriella was a prostitute who worked an area of the west side of Manhattan known as Hell's Kitchen, where I happened to live and work, too. Toothless and always dirty, she was not a pretty sight.

I often would see her on the corner of 43rd street, sometimes in a sleeping bag, as I hailed a cab to go to work in the morning. Recognizing one another, we'd often say hi. It was almost as though we hadn't punched in for our daytime jobs yet, for me to be her future doctor and for her to be my future patient.

Later, I would again often see her, agitated and suicidal at Roosevelt Hospital. She usually came in with a laceration, bleeding from a fight. These episodes were always linked with her cocaine and alcohol intoxication. It was hard to know what her baseline mental state was, since all our interactions, whether in the hospital or on the street, were a variation of hi and goodbye.

On one of her visits, a physician, who was more observant than I was, noticed her peculiar gait, which we had all been taking for granted. He had seen tabes dorsalis—the deterioration of part of the spinal cord due to syphilis—before and, given her professional promiscuity, wondered about neurological syphilis. Kicking and screaming, she was admitted, and we were soon able to get the needed tests done.

One such test involved sitting and talking with her long enough to realize how much we had been taking her for granted as just another person off the street. We found out that she was 47 years old and quite confused. Her short-term memory was poor, while her mood was quite grandiose and manic. She informed us that God had chosen her to bear the next baby Jesus. To our surprise, local street friends who knew her for years arrived to visit and filled in the blanks on her history. It was not one of mental illness or even, initially, drugs or alcohol, but that of a young pretty girl from a bad family who ran away from home into the street and never went back. They had noted significant changes in her mental state over the past year but attributed it to her alcohol and cocaine use.

It turned out she was not pregnant, but she did test positive for syphilis. There was more, as a CT of her head showed prominent ventricles. This is often a sign of atrophy or brain shrinkage found in many types of dementia and was clearly abnormal for her age. A lumbar puncture (spinal tap) was then done and the diagnosis was cinched. *Treponema pallidum* was present in Gabriella's cerebral spinal fluid, the liquid in, and surrounding, her brain. Gabriella had neurosyphilis.

Over the next year, through the help of some very creative social workers, we were able to rehabilitate Gabriella along with two other friends. We got them off the street and into stable housing with a focus on mental health and substance rehab. This allowed for continued medical treatment and monitoring of her infection. A year later she had recovered partially, but it was clear she would likely remain with some dementia and the scars of a very rough west side story for the rest of her life.

## A MODERN DAY PLAGUE

In the mid-80s, I was a medical student at the University of Miami when we began seeing cases of men with something new and very bad. No one knew what it was or what to do about it. All that was known to us in Miami, a gateway to the Third World, was that severe failure of the immune system was common to these cases and that it seemed to be happening in a select group. The word spread to watch out for the four H's—Haitian, hemophiliac, heroin, and homosexual. I remember how severely ill these patients were: their bodies bloated with edema; their lungs filled with foam, unable to breathe. The condition would soon be called call acquired immunodeficiency syndrome or AIDS and proven to be caused by a retrovirus called the human immunodeficiency virus or HIV.

The illness was transmitted through contact with bodily fluids, primarily blood but also semen. While intravenous drug users and those infected with blood products such as hemophiliacs, were initial primary targets, unprotected sex of any kind, but particularly in the Third World and especially between male homosexuals, impacted the greatest numbers.

To date, 30 million people worldwide have died of AIDS; two-thirds of those deaths occurred in Africa and were mostly acquired through unprotected sex in heterosexual situations. Currently there are as many people living with HIV, again with two-thirds in Africa. Half of all current African cases are women; one-tenth are under the age of 15.

In the United States, 1.7 million people have been infected with HIV and more than 600,000 deaths have occurred. Every year 40,000 males are diagnosed, compared with about 12,000 women. Male-to-male transmission accounts for 80 percent of infected men while 80 percent of women contract the virus through heterosexual activity. One in five of those infected with AIDS in the United States do not know they have it.

If there is a silver lining to all this, education about safe sex has curbed the rise of new cases. Additionally, a more aggressive treatment known as highly active antiretroviral therapy (HAART) has helped to turn the disease into a chronic one that people can live with rather than a death sentence. A significant reason for this turnaround is that the therapy ameliorates the effects the disease has on the central nervous system.

There was a time when 30 to 40 percent of cases would present with a neuropsychiatric symptom, such as depression, memory loss, or personality change. This was commonly the direct result of an inflammatory response the brain tissue was experiencing due to the presence of the HIV virus. This was not a good sign and predicted an aggressive course of the disease. Nowadays, the annual occurrence of AIDS dementia complex (ADC) is much lower because, in comparison to the past, many more people are aware of their HIV status and initiate early and aggressive treatment. At the same time, the overall numbers of ADC has risen. This is due to the now long-term nature of the disease; so many more people live with HIV-related problems.

In ADC, the neurological damage is thought to occur by virtue of an inflammatory response to the virus in the brain. Symptoms can vary from lethargy and apathy to memory loss and confusion. Mood issues are not uncommon, particularly depression and a personality change. Such was the case with Carl.

Carl was 46 years old when he was diagnosed with AIDS in 1998. The disease had presented with Kaposi's sarcoma, a skin lesion commonly found in AIDS patients. Carl was flabbergasted when the HIV test came back positive. "We were both in denial," said Ben, his lover who was also HIV positive. "He said he'd been safe, but when you're immersed in a culture of so many partners, something is bound to happen. When he came back positive I knew I'd be, too, because we were never safe together. We said we'd each get tested when we started out but just let it go, I think because we thought we'd be together forever. It didn't matter to me if I had it or not anymore. It was like we merged. Crazy, I know, but love does that. Honestly, I think I did get it from him. So here we are, still together, still with AIDS."

Ben was still relatively healthy when I met them while consulting at a nursing home. By then Carl was 57. Ben went on, thinking back, "I did well. Carl did too, for a while. We took our meds religiously, ate right, and got exercise. Work was good. We had lots of friends. Then, a few years ago, I began to see a change in him. It's hard to describe, kind of like the sparkle was gone. It was like someone turned off the light. His load had to be cut back at work—he lied to me about that until his boss told me. Our romantic life went into the toilet. He quit exercising and wouldn't go out. Stopping his meds was the worst thing because I know that's what accelerated all of this." I agreed with Carl, telling him that it has been established that the current antiviral therapy, HAART, is in part responsible for the decline in the incidence of HIV dementia. Ironically, the prevalence of HIV dementia is up because more people with the disease are living longer. As I told him, the situation is not unlike that of Alzheimer's: the more people that are living longer, the more that will experience dementia.

So Carl ended up in a nursing home with HIV-related dementia. His personality change had progressed into confusion and memory loss. He had recently been admitted to the hospital after going AWOL from Ben and winding up going from table to table, propositioning men, at a well-known gay bar. It was such a scene that an ambulance was called. From there Ben realized he could no longer care for his partner.

Ben and I found Carl alone in the common TV room watching a cartoon. Thin and drawn, he wore a cowboy hat. Before I could say a word, he told me he would not take any meds of any kind. Angry, depressed, and miserable, he was also confused and guarded and quite likely paranoid. I couldn't be sure what the reason was behind his refusal of medication. Looking at Ben, still quite healthy, I felt the disease had gotten hold of Carl long before he'd stopped his meds. So much is unknown about differences in our psychologies—our characters—and our immunity. Maybe that was why it was Carl who developed the dementia and not Ben. Carl kept his pledge not to take medications again for about another year. A short time later he died of pneumonia.

## FRONTOTEMPORAL DEMENTIA

The classic early onset or presenile dementia is called frontotemporal dementia (FTD). Second to early onset Alzheimer's disease, it accounts for about 20 percent of dementia in the earlier age groups.

FTD typically affects 40- to 65-year-olds but may occur in those as young as 20. The illness is aggressive. Many patients die in the first two to three years; the condition is almost 100 percent fatal after ten years. Specific atrophy, or shrinkage, of the frontal and then temporal lobes of the brain are the hallmark of the disease. This dementia was originally known as Pick's disease; however, variants of FTD have been identified.

The behavioral subtype remains more closely linked with the term Pick's disease. It is typified by a change in personality and a general apathy that usually predates any memory loss, thus clinically distinguishing it from Alzheimer's disease. Hoarding and gluttony can occur as well. This form of FTD can be genetically determined. A dysfunction of tau protein, which is intrinsic in the microtubule transport system between nerve cells in the brain, is common to this form. "Pick's bodies," seen under the microscope, are intracellular inclusions of tau protein and are markers of Pick's disease.

Other subtypes include one with a nonfluent aphasia, where the patient can no longer form sentences, and another with a fluent aphasia, where word finding or word recognition is the hallmark. The latter, also known as semantic FTD, is the least genetic form of the illness and the least related to classic Pick's disease.

John, who had the behavioral variant of FTD, was referred to us for inpatient hospitalization from the outpatient geriatric psychiatry clinic at the University of Washington. He was young, around 40, and already had the illness for a couple of years. His wife, Julie, and his teenage kids were devastated at the dramatic decline in this otherwise healthy engineer/marathon runner. Julie had been trying to manage him at home, but his inappropriate behavior was not meshing well with the teenagers, and particularly their friends. The effect was so severe that neither his son nor daughter was comfortable inviting anyone over. The friends had spread the word in school that John had touched them and made inappropriate comments. A few even said that he was a pervert. It was extremely embarrassing for his kids, as well as for Julie, who was forced to explain the situation to other parents.

Julie told me, "The whole thing turned me off to him. Finally I refused to have sex. It makes me feel like a participant in this circus. But at the same time it kills me because I love him so much. It's why we're here. I don't know where else to turn. I must go to work, and yet he can't be left alone. Besides, with his behaviors, who would stay with him? I don't think 'home' is going to work anymore."

Unfortunately, we had a terrible time with John, too. The behaviors became unmanageable soon after admission. He was strong and constantly fought with us, all the while refusing medications and any other help we offered. Eventually the family could no longer visit; his rage at them only heightened their distress. In only two weeks on our unit he went from a walking, talking, almost normal appearing guy to an intentionally sedated patient ready for palliative care.

Julie was understandably angry that things went this way. She had hoped that the hospital stay could turn things around. She certainly did not expect that her husband's condition would worsen. The hospitalization and all the associated changes were detrimental to John and her, as well their children, but there had been no other choice. Wanting him to be comfortable, she signed onto palliative care.

John was discharged to a memory care assisted living facility that never would have taken him without sedation. He actually thrived for a while and was able to go off palliative care, but he continued to deteriorate over the next year. He never returned home, and a couple of years later died from complications of his severe neurological disease.

## BRAIN INJURY

Technically, brain injury is not thought of as a form of dementia. However, it is so prevalent, and includes so many elements in common with dementia, that it deserves discussion here, particularly since sexual issues are often found in this group.

While there are differences between brain injury and classic dementia, there are similarities as well. Both dementia and brain injury involve anatomical damage to the brain. Perhaps the difference is whether or not the injury is progressive, which is the case for all forms of dementia. Brain injury, in contrast, is sudden. A car accident or a bullet can cause it. But there are aspects of dementia that are sudden, too. Consider a massive stroke. Granted, it is usually the culmination of multiple strokes that causes the dementia, but a big event may contribute as well: one large hemorrhage may easily leave a person in a state of dementia for life.

Plus, it's not as if brain injury can never be progressive. What about the progressive development of a fetus who will be born with a form of mental retardation? Or the progressive blows to the brain that Muhammad Ali took over the years that led to a state of what is now being called a Parkinson's dementia? It is well known that virtually any form of brain injury, from mental retardation to traumatic brain injury, will increase the risk of formally developing dementia later on. The brain injury from chronic alcohol abuse, sometimes called alcohol dementia of middle age, is also considered to be a risk factor for later dementia in old age. (See chapter 8)

A traumatic event, for example one caused by a penetrating object, can occur just about anywhere in the brain. It could be localized and involve one specific area that might affect sexual functioning, or it could be a global event and affect the entire brain. This is often the case with severe mental retardation or an anoxic episode where the brain is without oxygen for too long.

Sometimes, a bizarre brain injury will totally change a personality.

### *The Accidental Lobotomy*

On September 13, 1848, Phineas Gage, who was 25 years old, was working to build a railroad in Vermont. His job was to help pack charges of dynamite into rocks to break them up. He was known as a calm and responsible young man who did well at his job. Unfortunately, one charge went off while he was holding the packing rod near his head. The rod was blown through his cheek and out of the top of the front of his head, taking some of his frontal lobe with it. (The remains were found some 50 feet away.) Amazingly, Gage remained conscious and was transported to the hospital where he nearly died of an infection soon thereafter. He lived to be 38. The following is an account from Dr. Harlow, his physician, of his personality change:

> The equilibrium or balance, so to speak, between his intellectual faculties and animal propensities, seems to have been destroyed. He is fitful, irreverent, indulging at times in the grossest profanity (which was not previously his custom), manifesting but little deference for his fellows, impatient of restraint or advice when it conflicts with his desires, at times pertinaciously obstinate, yet capricious and vacillating, devising many plans of future operations, which are no sooner arranged than they are abandoned in turn for others appearing more feasible. A child in his intellectual capacity and manifestations, he has the animal passions of a strong man. Previous to his injury, although untrained in the schools, he possessed a well-balanced mind, and was looked upon by those who knew him as a shrewd, smart businessman, very energetic and

> persistent in executing all his plans of operation. In this regard his mind was radically changed, so decidedly that his friends and acquaintances said he was "no longer Gage."

The damage in Gage's brain, with his subsequent personality change, profanities, and vulgarities has been the subject of medical and neurological discussion ever since. While his brain rests in a museum, parallels continue to be made between his case and more contemporary neurological phenomena. A recent report by Jack van Horn, a UCLA assistant professor of neurology, and colleagues noted that while approximately 4 percent of the cerebral cortex was intersected by the rod's passage, more than 10 percent of Gage's total white matter was damaged. The passage of the tamping iron caused widespread damage to the white matter connections throughout Gage's brain, which likely was a major contributor to the behavioral changes he experienced. The press release from UCLA regarding the report included the following:

- "The extensive loss of white matter connectivity, affecting both hemispheres, plus the direct damage by the rod, which was limited to the left cerebral hemisphere, is not unlike modern patients who have suffered a traumatic brain injury," he [Van Horn] said. "And it is analogous to certain forms of degenerative diseases, such as Alzheimer's disease or frontal temporal dementia, in which neural pathways in the frontal lobes are degraded, which is known to result in profound behavioral changes."
- Van Horn noted that the quantification of the changes to Gage's brain's pathways might well provide important insights for clinical assessment and outcome-monitoring in modern-day brain trauma patients.

### *The Age of the Lobotomy*

Accidental brain piercing resulting in personality change is one thing. Removing parts of a person's brain on purpose is something else entirely. Still, anthropologic and archeological findings reveal that an intentional surgical procedure appears to have been performed in various places around the world dating to before the time of Christ. However, it wasn't until the turn of the 20th century that such procedures were considered for modern medical purposes.

Pioneered by the neurologist António Moniz in Portugal in the 1930s, this psychosurgery took the form of the frontal lobotomy and was intended to be used for uncontrolled or debilitating behaviors, as well as intractable pain. Patients ranged from those with severe depression to schizophrenics and those with dementia. The procedure was even performed on those with sexual disorders, the definition of which was open to interpretation. Homosexuality, for example, was considered a pathologic condition by the *Diagnostic and Statistical Manual of Mental Disorders* (the primary reference tool used by psychiatrists even today) well into the 1970s. I am aware of reports of girls getting lobotomies to be more complaisant with sexual abuse, and an account of a wife for whom a lobotomy was surreptitiously used to make her comply with ongoing abuse between her husband and their daughter.

In 1945, neuropsychiatrist Walter Freeman and neurosurgeon Richard Watts began experimenting with a simpler procedure than drilling two holes through either side of the skull and inserting a blade to transect the frontal lobe. Freeman, playing with an ice pick and a grapefruit in his kitchen, developed the new procedure. A "refined" technique was soon applied regularly by inserting a six-inch long pick-like instrument up into the tissue above each eye ball. A mallet was used to tap on the instrument, break through the bone at the back of the eye socket, and enter the brain. Moving the pick from side to side, the connections within the frontal lobe were then severed.

Based upon the negative personality changes seen in Phineas Gage, one might wonder why the frontal lobotomy was used in the first place. The answer seems to be that the separation of any mindfulness or planning over such core emotions as sexuality appears to have taken precedence over the lack of impulse control and disinhibition that occurred as a common side effect. Other side effects were also common, including severe personality changes, cognitive damage, seizures, and even death. These were often associated with unexpected bleeding or infection.

The discovery of antipsychotics greatly curtailed the use of lobotomy in the early 1950s, but not before some 50,000 people received the procedure. Moniz won the Nobel Prize in Physiology or Medicine in 1949 for developing the lobotomy.

Today, dramatic head injuries leading immediately to a dementia-like state occur on a regular basis. Common causes include gunshot or blast injuries either at war or at home, car accidents, and even failed suicide attempts. All of these may have sexual side effects associated with them.

Mitch, for instance, was a quiet man who tended to isolate himself from others. He struggled with depression his entire life and his father and brother had killed themselves. According to the family, he was diagnosed with dementia in 2002 but had been doing fairly well. His niece looked in on Mitch, who lived close by in a small mountain community near Mount Rainier. But one morning in 2004, without warning, Mitch raised a pistol to the side of his head and pulled the trigger.

"I guess I pointed the gun wrong," he told me two months later when I met him. "But I'm glad I didn't kill myself." I was glad for that as well, as I inspected the face of this man who had literally blown off the entire frontal lobe of his brain. One could easily see that something was missing. The surgeons had apparently just put a plate in, pulled the skin back and stitched it up. Of course, I was seeing him in part to assess his potential for further suicidality, which he may have cured by lobotomizing himself. Still, some odd behaviors had been noted in Mitch. He was found to be impulsive with his words and actions. The mostly female staff members were facing the challenge of keeping his provocative comments under control and were looking for guidance on how to handle him. Complicating matters, neither Mitch nor his family was interested in any psychiatric management, medication or otherwise. This limited my involvement to an educational discussion with the staff about the frontal lobe syndrome, which he clearly had. He was discharged soon thereafter and returned to the mountains to be closer to family. I never saw or heard from him again.

## DEMENTIA PUGILISTICA

In June 2007, Chris Benoit, a 40-year-old wrestler, killed his wife and child and then himself. An autopsy revealed his brain to have changes similar to those found in Alzheimer's disease. At least three deceased National Football League (NFL) players have been diagnosed with, or showed strong evidence of, chronic traumatic encephalopathy (CTE). Mike Webster, Terry Long, and Andre Waters died, respectively, at ages 50, 42, and 44. Long and Waters committed suicide. Waters' brain resembled that of an octogenarian with Alzheimer's disease. All these men suffered from dementia pugilistica.

Dementia puglistica is a syndrome most commonly associated with boxing. However, recent attention has been focused on several sports involving repeat head concussions. Football, from professional to Pee Wee, finally appears to be taking a center stage position. There is a buzz over lawsuits, helmet changes, and even rule changes such as the consideration to take the high impact kick-off out of the NFL.

It is well known that personality changes are commonly a part of the syndrome. Manic behavior, including hypersexuality, inappropriate demands, and a Klüver–Bucy–like syndrome have been described. I experienced such a case at our inpatient service in 2010.

Shorty was a 60-year-old ex-boxer with a Parkinson's-like syndrome tremor and slowed gait. He felt that these symptoms were associated with his years of repeated trauma to his brain. Most recently he had developed some strange moods characterized by elation, along with sexual advances to women in restaurants. This behavior had become an embarrassment to Kate, his wife, after she witnessed it several times.

"This is not him. I don't understand what is going on," she told me. "His memory has been bad. He doesn't listen to me. And now this behavior with the women is going on. His doctor told me the Parkinson's stuff was because he fought until he was 38, but I never expected this. How could this happen all these years after stopping? Don't tell me it's Alzheimer's."

I explained that her husband's symptoms were a common combination of trauma and time. A younger brain may well be able to absorb the battering without symptoms, but later, as the brain ages, the damage is still there. "Brain trauma is a well-known risk for Alzheimer's but I've always felt that brain damage itself and age is more the issue," I told her.

Careful history taking often reveals more deficit than is initially presented. I discovered that Shorty really hadn't been all that functional sexually, or even that interested in sex, for years. He'd been unable to hold down a job. His wife drove the car and handled the finances. She worked as a real estate broker while he stayed home and did chores that she assigned to him. Interestingly, the neurologists were about to put Shorty on Parkinson's medication, which, with their dopamine punch, would have made him much worse sexually than he was. We opted to hold off on that until we could get his behaviors under better control. He responded well to a mood stabilizer and was released back to his wife with a follow-up appointment to a neurologist.

And then there was the case of Gil, who, at 55, was admitted to us for aggressive behavior. Gil clearly had a cognitive deficit consistent with dementia and had been diagnosed by the military as suffering with CTE. He presented to our inpatient service directly from an office visit at Madigan Army Hospital. He had taken many blast injuries after several tours in the Middle East.

His wife, Laura, was depressed. She said, "This violence has got to stop. They don't seem to be able to control it. It has ruined him. It has ruined us." As it turned out, Gil and Laura had been struggling with his violence for years. She had called the police multiple times for domestic violence. Each time he was taken to jail and each time she would end up picking him up. "I am done with this, I just can't do this to myself anymore," she told me.

We were able to get him stable with some medication, but she was right; the long-term picture really was dependent upon their living apart. With help from the army, we were able to get Gil into a long-term program to help stabilize each of them. I discovered about a year later that, for better or worse, Laura had taken him back home again.

We often think of brain trauma as a blast or bullet or blow. Yet there are other events that can be equally devastating to the brain tissue. One of my most memorable cases involved two friends, the right intention, and a bad situation.

## LIFE AFTER CARDIAC ARREST

Bo, 46, was a volunteer fireman in a small town in eastern Washington State. He and his best friend, Ned, also 46, met with the other volunteers each Wednesday night to practice their lifesaving and firefighting skills. They both enjoyed sounding off the local alarm, the signal that it was meeting night at the firehouse, that blasted through the community. After the meeting they would usually go over to one or the other's home for a couple of beers.

Each fireman was equipped with a radio signal device that could transmit an alarm from the station in the middle of the night when the loud community siren was not practical. One night Ned was awakened by the bedside tone, which was always followed by the address of the call. This one was especially ominous; it was Bo's house.

Ned raced there and was the first to arrive. Bo's wife, Lillie, along with their children, ran out in terror onto the front lawn, screaming that Bo was unconscious on the kitchen floor. Ned told me later that he knew it would be bad because no resuscitative efforts had been started by Lillie, who was hysterical. Bo was blue and completely arrested. Precious minutes had passed. Ned started with some deep breaths into Bo's lungs and then began compressions. More breaths. More compressions. Finally, he heard sirens. Help was there.

Given the time that had passed, the EMTs defibrillated Bo immediately. To Ned's amazement, the flat line suddenly showed a rhythm, slow at first but then faster. Soon there was shallow breathing, and then deeper breaths. Ned walked out into the front yard and hugged Lillie.

"We saved him. He's alive."

"Thank God," Lillie sobbed. But Ned silently wondered about his friend's condition. Too many minutes had passed without oxygen.

Bo was in the hospital for 45 days. He was first placed in the ICU and then moved to a step-down, where the focus gradually changed from his heart to his brain. He was in a coma for a week and then gradually awoke. But he was foggy and emotional. He became agitated, then flat. He didn't recognize anyone. The neurologist ordered tests, including an EEG, which showed slow waves, a potential sign that the brain was damaged. Yet there was room for hope that with more rehabilitation and time, Bo would recover.

I met them all during his second hospitalization, about three months after the cardiac arrest. As it turned out, Bo's father had died of a heart attack at 49. "He was there one minute and gone the next," Ned explained. Things were turning out differently for Bo. He had gone to a rehab and was able to make eye contact but not able to walk. Then came episodes of agitation, anger, and then giddiness with more and more sexually inappropriate behavior. Rude comments, solicitation of every woman he saw, and grabbing the staff were now his norm. The rehab made it clear that he couldn't stay unless he was evaluated and treated.

By then, Ned and Lillie realized that Bo's brain damage was permanent. Lillie, however, was not ready to give up and became angry with the idea that he might now have dementia. We treated Bo somewhat successfully with mood stabilizing medication, but the rehab never took him back. He eventually went to a small adult family home where there were only men. Bo, unlike his wife and best friend, went out smiling, having forgotten everything that happened to him.

But Ned was another story. He took me aside and asked for some Xanax, explaining that he couldn't sleep. "It's entirely my fault," he said. I asked why he would say such a thing. He replied, "I knew he was down for too long without oxygen, but I don't know what I could have done differently. The result of oxygen-depletion is permanent. Irreversible damage starts after about four minutes. If he could see himself, with this embarrassing behavior in front of his wife and daughters, it would kill him. I know this man. He'd rather be dead."

## POSTTRAUMATIC STRESS DISORDER

A review of the literature relating to posttraumatic stress disorder (PTSD) found that dementia is related to a resurgence of PTSD symptoms. While these patients primarily suffered with war-related PTSD, I have seen sexually related regressive phenomena as well. In particular, there can be a resurgence of emotional reactions to child sexual abuse or adult rape. An Australian newsletter discusses this relatively unexplored area. It mentions the high probability of expression of unresolved childhood sexual trauma in the one in four females and one in six boys who develop dementia later in life. Considering that the Australian numbers for dementia are similar to that of the United States—one-third of 80-year-olds—this is a substantial issue. I have dealt with cases of the disorder myself.

I met Guy and Crystal on our inpatient unit, where she was hospitalized for dementia with depression. Guy shared with me the details of her difficult life. Crystal was a beautiful girl, but between the ages of 12 and 14, she was repeatedly molested by her grandfather. This changed her and led to a life of mistrust, in particular of men.

"She never really trusted me completely, but I am just so easygoing and getting married was the thing to do. I guess she figured it would be me," Guy told me. "We moved to Idaho where I worked with my dad in a small town, but all the women despised her looks, which made it all worse. So we moved from there, had our kids, and over the years just kind of swept it all under the rug. Romantically, I always knew when to back off, but she respected my sexual needs, too.

"Then came the dementia. It was like dumping salt back on the wound. She started living the abuse all over again and got paranoid. She thought I was having an affair. We've been struggling with that ever since with antipsychotics and hospitalizations. That abuse just made her dementia a mess. I still love her. I wish she could love me."

PTSD doesn't just pop up out of nowhere. It's a known entity that is present when the relationship starts, if not overtly then with symptoms of mistrust. The symptoms will become reinflamed as the years of healing and sealing over fade away, leaving the raw memories exposed once again. For the partner it's a matter of love, commitment, and belief that the spouse with dementia still loves him or her. Simply being there, through treatments that very likely could involve medications and hospitalizations, is most important. For the patient, there is nothing that can be said that will change the horrible memories that have become a part of who they are. It is unfortunate that these thoughts are so often connected to the longer-term memories that are so often preserved long into the course of the dementia.

## TOUGH CHOICES

Additional causes of other dementias include purely genetic dementing illnesses, such as Huntington's disease (HD) or familial Creutzfeldt-Jakob disease (CJD), which bring difficult reproductive decisions to the table. In such cases a young man or woman who knows he or she has a 50 percent chance of carrying the gene for a disease that will eventually kill them (HD sooner than CJD) must make very tough decisions. They need to decide whether they want to know their own fate and if they want to risk passing the gene on to their children. It's a very difficult scenario, and one I've seen played out.

Wanda and her boyfriend Keith watched as we struggled in the care facility to get her 45-year-old father down onto the bed and give him something to calm him. Suffering from HD, he showed all the markers of the condition: involuntary flailing movements of his arms and legs, confusion, and erratic behavior. On this day, he grabbed a nurse around the neck so hard she had to be admitted to the hospital. The day before he cornered a social worker and seized her breasts.

Having seen the symptoms evolve over the past 10 years, none of this behavior was new to Wanda. Keith, on the other hand, looked stricken. I had a chance to speak with them after things had calmed down.

"I wanted you to see this, Keith," she began. "This is why, if we get married, we cannot have kids." Turning to me, she explained that she had already told Keith that there was a 50 percent chance she carried the gene. If that was the case, there was a 50 percent chance that each of their children would have the gene, not to mention there would be a 100 percent chance she would get the disease later. I asked her if she had considered getting tested so she would know one way or the other.

"I'm 25. I have been thinking about that test for years. It's like gambling. If it's negative, I breathe a sigh of relief. If it's positive, I'll be like my dad. Some people couldn't take it and would have to know. I'd rather find out later."

I looked at Keith. Still a little shaken, he just shrugged his shoulders and sighed.

CHAPTER EIGHT

# The Sexual Effects of Delirium, Drugs, and Other Substances

There is another class of brain malfunction closely linked to dementia and commonly associated with changes in sexuality. Delirium is the medical term used for acute brain failure and may also be associated with other mental symptoms, such as a decreased level of alertness or wakefulness, often called a "clouding of consciousness," which may fluctuate. Visual hallucinations, unstable moods, or a personality change are also possible.

As opposed to dementia, where there is generally progressive destruction of brain tissue over months to years, delirium is an adverse stimulation to the brain that often takes hold over hours to days. There is usually not a permanent destruction of brain tissue but rather a reversible assault on the physiology and function of the brain that, if left alone, may quickly lead to death.

Drugs and certain substances aside, the adverse stimuli causing delirium may be just about anything one can imagine that changes the circumstances under which the brain operates. These include toxins from infections and fevers, as well as changes in blood chemistry, such as a high sugar level or a change in oxygen levels. Water, too, in high enough quantities, can cause it. An environmental change, such as an extended stay in an ICU or a sudden change to new surroundings, may also lead to delirium.

One of the most common causes of delirium in the elderly, as well as in dementia patients, is a urinary tract infection (UTI). This is much more commonly associated with increased confusion and lethargy than any sexual symptoms. On occasion, however, it might make itself known with changes in heightened sexuality. UTIs are most likely to be a bladder infection in woman and prostatitis in men. In either case, there may be a sensation of incomplete bladder emptying, burning, or other sensitivity. In confused patients unable to understand or discuss what is bothering them, these symptoms may be associated with increased focus on the genitals.

Even the time of day might have an effect on the functioning of a brain made sensitive enough through the changes of dementia. Sundowning, just like delirium, is a worsening of confusion seen in dementia patients when the sun goes down. In reality, this change may occur much closer to noon in some patients and may last through the night in others. It remains unclear what actually causes this phenomenon, but it is generally felt to be more associated with our internal clock rather than whether the sun is up or down. It is thought that sundowning may be due to dementia-related injury to the specialized area of the brain, the suprachiasmatic nucleus in the hypothalamus, which helps to regulate that clock.

## A JEKYLL/HYDE CASE

Years ago, I treated, in the hospital, a woman named Louise. She exhibited dementia-related sexual behaviors specific to the afternoon and evening. It seems that every afternoon she would become unmanageable at her memory care assisted living facility due to her constant sexual propositioning of men. This was one of the most dramatic cases of sundowning I've ever seen because of her ability to describe, in the morning, what was going to happen in the afternoon.

"I was raised in Wyoming," I remember her explaining in a frightened voice. "We'd see the shadows come across the plains as the thunderstorms built and moved with the shifting wind. That's what it's like for me. I know it's going to happen every day, just after lunch. The shadow catches up with me, and it all changes. I'm scared."

And then, over the course of an hour or so, she'd be gone, changed like a female version of Dr. Jekyll and Mr. Hyde. A formerly frightened and cowering individual was now very confidently asking me to engage with her in certain sexual activities. No longer was I just her doctor. Now I was a handsome man and likely a good kisser, too.

### *Clouded Consciousness in Action*

Although classic delirium is described as a clouding of consciousness, in practice this may be a very late stage of the process whereby other mental or neurological changes might be noticed earlier. Recognizing the delirium early could have an impact on the outcome.

Take, for example, acute alcohol intoxication, a common form of delirium. It's Friday, 6:00 p.m., and the evening is just getting started. The first drink arrives and, maybe half an hour later, the second. Delirium is setting in, yet there is no clouding of consciousness. In fact, the opposite—giddy, energetic, disinhibited behavior—is usually the case. By the third drink, depending on the person, the neurological motor symptoms of slightly slurred speech, poor coordination, and less steady gait begin. Only later will a clouding of consciousness—in this case, sleepiness—begin.

## MEDICATIONS AND SEXUAL SYMPTOMS IN DEMENTIA

A member of a dementia support group sent me this email:

> *My husband was diagnosed with dementia a few years ago and currently takes donepezil and Namenda as well as lisinopril for his blood pressure. His memory is okay but he gets confused and has trouble making decisions and plans. I thought we were managing well but now, after over a decade of impotence, he wants to resume our sex life! And his doctor gave him a prescription for Viagra! That chapter of my life is over and I am just not interested, but he keeps pressuring me and I don't know what to do.*

This is a classic dementia drug interaction case. As far as the medications go, four are mentioned: Aricept (donepezil), Namenda, Viagra, and lisinopril. My first thought when I read the posting was, what is the point of his being on aggressive treatment of his dementia with two medications (Aricept and Namenda), if he isn't allowed to fully live his life? He might want the computer for pornography, since there doesn't appear to be much going on in the bedroom.

This medication scenario is common to sex and dementia. The Aricept and Namenda are likely in part responsible for his even being able to have the sexual desires he feels. They work to keep his cognition stable. There is ample evidence that the activity of acetylcholine promotes erection, and Aricept works by increasing the presence of this neurotransmitter. He still may not be getting an erection, but it is possible it is helping him along. The Viagra, of course, is for erections and could likely be successful for him. Lisinopril, prescribed for high blood pressure, is a common medication notorious for causing sexual dysfunction. The use of this drug must be balanced with the medical risks of uncontrolled high blood pressure. Before adding the Viagra, his doctor could have considered adjusting the dosage of the lisinopril first.

There are many prescribed medications associated with sexual symptoms (see the box "Medications with Sexual Side Effects," later in this chapter), many of which are used in dementia patients. Those that are sedating, such as hypnotic benzodiazepines or the narcotics, will contribute to a lessening of sexual activity. These two classes of medications are known to cause delirium, however, which would be associated with heightened sexual activity.

All antipsychotics will lessen sexual activity, and one of the most common side effects of antidepressants—especially the selective serotonin inhibitors—is sexual inhibition. This is because serotonin tends to calm anxiety and improve mood, but it also tends to take away one's sexual desire. That's what happened to Tammy.

Bob and Tammy had been best friends, lovers, and devoted husband and wife for 50 years. Nothing was going to stop them, certainly not the dementia that Tammy had been diagnosed with about a year before I met him at an Alzheimer's conference. Bob approached me after my talk and asked about Paxil. Tammy had been placed on this well-known selective serotonin reuptake inhibitor (SSRI) antidepressant about six months previously for depression or, as Bob put it, "a sort of disinterest in things. She got better in some ways but you talked about sex during your lecture and that was always our strong point. Her mood came back, but that went away."

Listening to Bob, I immediately suspected the problem was with the Paxil. As I knew their primary doctor, I offered to give him a call.

When the physician and I spoke about Bob and Tammy, we talked about two contemporary antidepressants, Wellbutrin (buproprion) and Remeron (mirtazapine), that are commonly used in the elderly.

Given that Tammy was also having trouble maintaining her weight, the primary doctor stopped the Paxil and switched her to a low dose of Remeron, which is a great appetite stimulant. I followed up with the doctor a month later, and I was relieved to learn that Tammy was eating well, her mood remained good, and things were back to normal sexually.

Stimulants are sometimes used for depression in dementia patients. While they decrease appetite, they may increase sexual desire, even obsessive/compulsive sexual behaviors, due to their augmentation of dopamine activity. However, they will always worsen sexual performance. The same is true of many of the Parkinson's medications, again due to increased dopamine activity. These include Sinemet (carbidopa-levodopa), Mirapex (pramipexole), Requip (ropinirole), Eldepryl (selegiline), and Pergolide (bromocriptine). Tom's case was a textbook illustration of the effects of Parkinson's medications.

## CAUGHT BETWEEN A NURSE AND A HARD PLACE

Tom had suffered with Parkinson's disease for years when I first met him and his wife, Madge, in an assisted living facility. She had placed him there due to his dementia and care needs and was concerned that he was depressed. Tom ate a little breakfast and then slept the rest of the day.

Madge was a retired surgical nurse with a take-charge personality to match. She wanted Tom's mood to improve ASAP, but at the same time gave me a very long list of all the antidepressants he'd been on over the years. None, it seemed, gave any benefit. Her opinion was that all the psych drugs had hastened the development of both his Parkinson's and his dementia. Yet despite her frustration with his meds, she was convinced that selegiline would be the perfect choice for him. Her argument was that it would activate him, giving him stamina and vigor while helping to strengthen the activity of his current Parkinson's medications. Then she presented her proof: her friend's husband had taken it, and he was much improved.

I, on the other hand, was not convinced that selegiline was the way to go. We discussed the possibility of overactivating him in his fragile state. Madge saw the situation differently. Her reply was, "Exactly."

Tom was put on the drug and, for a week or so, did well. His Parkinson's symptoms seemed to loosen up, and his mood was better.

But then the problems began. At first Tom was up at night, and he wandered. Then he began flirting with the staff, who also noted that he was masturbating in his room. When Madge arrived he either demanded from one minute to the next that she take him home, or insisted that she have sex with him.

After a number of days, it was clear that he had gone into a hyperexcited manic-like state that, with the tremendous anxiety it generated, was uncomfortable for him and everyone else around him. He was taken off the selegiline, and a couple of days later he had calmed down. His Parkinson's symptoms, however, slipped back and downward, as did his affect—his ability to relate emotionally. Others noted as well that his mood wasn't as much an issue as his mask-life demeanor. I was finally able to convince Madge of that, and Tom's treatment proceeded more conservatively from that point. Tom lived another year or so with the two of them able to spend quality time together and share some good memories. She seemed less distressed by his illness, which I realized later had been the motivation that drove her to help him.

## THE TRICYCLICS AND TRAZADONE

The older antidepressants developed during the 1960s, such as Elavil (amitriptyline) or Sinequan (doxepin), are sometimes prescribed for dementia patients as a sleep aid. Many are tricyclics, named after their three-ringed biochemical form. Elavil is used in low doses for pain as well. These drugs can be very anticholinergic, that is, they block the acetylcholine. The result includes dry mouth, blurred vision, constipation, and urine retention. The drugs also have a sedating effect, as well as causing confusion. Given these side effects, they are of little use to the elderly or those with dementia.

Trazadone, a four-ringed antidepressant developed in the 1960s, has less toxic effects overall and is still used today to treat dementia patients. It causes fewer of the anticholinergic side effects, yet retains sedation properties. Unlike other sedative-hypnotics, the drug tends to be well tolerated and is not habit forming. However, it does have one significant side effect that, at times, may go unnoticed. That's what happened in one patient's case.

George, whose diagnosis was mild dementia, was in a nursing home when I met him. Because he was experiencing a lot of trouble with sleep he was given 50 milligrams of Elavil nightly. This is fine if it works and is tolerated, but in George's case it was neither. He wasn't sleeping well and suffered with a very dry mouth and urine retention.

I stopped the Elavil and put him on Trazadone. He slept much better and seemed to tolerate the drug well. Then, a week later, I was called because of George's inappropriate sexual behavior. It turned out that he had an erection when a nurse entered his room. To me, the reaction seemed naïve and overreactive as sex happens in nursing homes, and it was likely that the nurse had entered at an unfortunate time. The director of nursing agreed with me. But then the incident happened again the next day, and it quickly became apparent that George had a continuous erection that was being interpreted as sexual in nature.

As I was not available to see him, I asked the nursing director to speak to George. As she later related to me, he had been trying to hide the erection. To him, it was anything but sexual, and he was in physical pain. Both the nursing director and I knew that the situation was alarming.

Priapism is a relatively uncommon pathologic erection of the penis. It is, however, considered a medical emergency as it may lead to destruction of the penile tissue and even require amputation. (Women taking Trazadone may also experience priapism with clitoral erections, but there is a much lower incidence of this.) Although priapism related to Trazadone is relatively uncommon, it is a serious complication that may go unnoticed due to patient embarrassment and staff misinterpretation.

George was sent to the hospital for immediate treatment. Fortunately, he responded to medical therapy that involved injecting an adrenaline-like agent into the penis to counter the antiadrenaline action of the Trazadone. The smooth muscle in the penis must be relaxed to obtain an erection. Adrenaline acts to contract the smooth muscle. Thus its presence is not conducive to having an erection. This is one reason why anxiety or drug stimulants are not conducive to sexual performance in men.

As for George, he was placed on melatonin to help him sleep, and it worked for him.

## SEX HORMONES AND DEMENTIA

Libido is stimulated by testosterone in men and women. It is also known that testosterone levels—most dramatically in men—drop in later life. This decline has been implicated as a potential cause in some dementia cases. Despite the obvious inclination to use testosterone as a more formal treatment for dementia, doing so has never become popular due, in part, to controversy over the long-term health consequences of testosterone replacement in elderly men.

Estrogen replacement therapy (ERT) has found a place with many older women, although it too has been linked with health risks, including certain cancers, thus stirring controversy. Still, brain health in particular seems to benefit, as do some negative sexual aspects of menopause such as decreased libido in some women.

However, other studies demonstrate that testosterone is the driving hormonal force behind libido and that estrogen replacement, with or without progesterone, has little benefit relative to loss of sexual desire. Nonetheless, estrogen therapy does help to maintain a healthy vaginal mucosa leading to less infectious and inflammatory complications related to sexual activity in elderly women.

For men, the estrogen situation is different. Studies report that elderly men taking this hormone have shown increased serious medical complications, such as stroke and cardiac events. There is also a clear suppression of testosterone from this therapy and thus a suppression of sexual activity and performance as shown in studies on male to female transsexuals.

Depo-Provera (medroxyprogesterone acetate), a well-known female contraceptive, is a form of synthetic progesterone. It is also used to treat breast cancer and endometriosis and has been shown to have an inhibitory effect on sexual behavior in men through its suppression of testosterone activity. It has been used for chemical castration in sexual offenders, as well as limiting the sexual activity of men with dementia who are unresponsive to other forms of treatment for inappropriate sexual behavior.

HAART (highly active antiretroviral therapy) has revolutionized the treatment of HIV disease, rendering it a chronic illness rather than a death sentence. Despite new concerns, such as an increased prevalence of AIDS dementia complex as a result of longer viral presence in the people living with AIDS for many years, studies show that there has not been an increase of higher-risk sexual behavior with HARRT. There is, in fact, some evidence that HAART itself may be directly associated with sexual dysfunction.

## *Medications with Sexual Side Effects*

**Prescription Medications**

Other than impotence and ejaculatory problems, both men and women experience all the side effects.

| Antidepressants | Main Use | Possible Effect on Sexual Function |
|---|---|---|
| MAOI antidepressants (Nardil, Parnate) | Depression | Decreased sex drive, impotence, delayed orgasm |
| SSRI antidepressants (Celexa, Lexapro, Paxil, Prozac, Zoloft) | Depression, anxiety | Decreased sex drive, impotence, delayed or absent orgasm, ejaculatory disturbances |
| SRI antidepressants (Cymbalta, Effexor) | Depression, anxiety | Same as above |
| Tricyclic antidepressants (amitriptyline, doxepin Tofranil) | Depression | Same as above |
| Clonidine | High blood pressure | Impotence, decreased sex drive, delayed or failure of ejaculation |
| Methyldopa | High blood pressure | Impotence, decreased sex drive, ejaculatory failure |
| Thiazide diuretics (e.g., bendroflumethiazide) | High blood pressure | Impotence, decreased sex drive |
| **Antiepileptics** | **Main Use** | **Possible Effect on Sexual Function** |
| Carbamazepine | Epilepsy | Impotence |
| **Antihypertensives** | **Main Use** | **Possible Effect on Sexual Function** |
| ACE inhibitors (lisinopril, enalapril) | High blood pressure, heart failure | Impotence |

*(continued)*

***Medications with Sexual Side Effects (continued)***

| **Antihypertensives *(continued)*** | **Main Use** | **Possible Effect on Sexual Function** |
|---|---|---|
| Alpha-blockers (doxazosin, prazosin) | High blood pressure, enlarged prostate | Impotence, ejaculatory disturbances |
| Beta-blockers (atenolol, propranolol, timolol eye drops) | High blood pressure, angina, glaucoma | Impotence |
| Calcium channel blockers (nifedipine, verapamil) | High blood pressure, angina | Impotence |

| **Antipsychotics** | **Main Use** | **Possible Effect on Sexual Function** |
|---|---|---|
| *Typical** | | |
| Haldol, Thorazine | Psychotic illness | Ejaculatory disturbances, decreased sex drive, impotence |
| *Atypical* | | |
| Risperdal, Seroquel, Zyprexa (most used) | Bipolar and psychotic illness | Same as above |
| Abilify, Clozaril, Geodon, Invega | Same as above | Same as above |

*Typical antipsychotics are older versions of the drugs versus the atypicals, or newer versions. The best-known typicals include Haldol (haloperidol) and Thorazine (chlorpromazine). Their packaging does not include black box warnings (literally a warning inside a black box on the label) about increased risk of death in dementia patients. The typicals tend to cause more side effects than the newer atypicals, which is why the latter are used more often. The most well-known atypicals include Risperdal (risperidone), Seroquel (quetiapine), and Zyprexa (olanzapine). Their packaging does include black box warnings.

| **Cholesterol-Lowering Medicines** | **Main Use** | **Possible Effect on Sexual Function** |
|---|---|---|
| Fibrates (e.g., clofibrate, gemfibrozil) | High cholesterol | Impotence |
| Statins (e.g., simvastin) | High cholesterol | Impotence |

*(continued)*

*Medications with Sexual Side Effects (continued)*

| Parkinson's Disease Medications | Main Use | Possible Effect on Sexual Function |
|---|---|---|
| Eldepryl, Mirapex, Pergolide, Requip, Sinemet | Parkinson's symptoms, restless legs | Increased libido, erectile dysfunction, anorgasmia |
| **Other** | **Main Use** | **Possible Effect on Sexual Function** |
| Benzodiazepines (e.g., Ativan, Xanax) | Anxiety, insomnia | Decreased sex drive |
| Cimetidine | Peptic ulcers, acid reflux disease | Decreased sex drive, impotence |
| Cyproterone acetate | Prostate cancer | Decreased libido, impotence, reduced volume of ejaculation |
| Disulfiram | Alcohol withdrawal | Decreased sex drive, impotence |
| Finasteride | Enlarged prostate | Decreased sex drive, ejaculation disorders, reduced volume of ejaculation |
| Metoclopramide | Nausea, vomiting | Decreased sex drive, impotence |
| Omeprazole | Peptic ulcers, acid reflux disease | Impotence |
| Opioid pain killers (e.g., Fentanyl, morphine, OxyContin, Vicodin) | Severe pain | Decreased sex drive, impotence |
| Prochlorperazine | Nausea, vomiting | Impotence |
| Propantheline | Gut spasm | Increased libido, impotence, anorgasmia |
| Stimulants (amphetamine, Ritalin) | Attention deficit hyperactivity disorder (ADHD), depression | Impotence |

*(continued)*

*Medications with Sexual Side Effects (continued)*

| Over-the-Counter Medications | |
|---|---|
| Antihistamine/decongestants (diphenhydramine [Benadryl], cetirizine [Zyrtec]) | Decreased libido |
| Pain medications (acetaminophen, aspirin, ibuprofen) | Erectile dysfunction |

## SUBSTANCE ABUSE AND DEMENTIA

Many substances have been implicated as causal agents in dementia. Who hasn't heard a story about a glue-sniffing teenager whose brain was destroyed? Yet having been involved in the treatment of well over 20,000 cases of dementia, I have yet to meet this person or anyone like him. Similar substances, such as industrial solvents, have been cited as well. While there is no doubt that these substances are neurotoxic and could damage the brain, the practical reality is that there are just not many cases reported in industrialized countries.

There are also many street drugs that have been implicated as potentially being a cause in the development of dementia: Heroin, LSD, cocaine, methamphetamine, and marijuana are the usual suspects. Of these, cocaine and methamphetamine, because of their stimulant properties, have been implicated in stroke disease and thus in the development of dementia through either acute or chronic abuse. Additionally, other types of pre-dementias are thought to be accelerated by the use of these substances, although the mechanism of this remains unclear.

Both cocaine and methamphetamine act, in part, by augmenting the action of dopamine, which is linked to hypersexual and compulsive behaviors (see chapter 3). This mechanism, with the potential for creation of manic states through dopamine and the effects on other neurotransmitters, such as serotonin and adrenalin, can produce any number of augmented sexual scenarios. To the extent that those with HIV or stroke disease, with already compromised brains, abuse these substances, it is quite possible that such scenarios are all the more heightened and even a reason for repetitious abuse.

Mr. H (as he preferred to be addressed) was a 61-year-old who often frequented the psychiatric emergency service in the New York

City hospital I worked in. He would most often be brought in by emergency medical services (EMS) for behaviors he exhibited on the street. Once in a while, he would be brought in for sexual behaviors, such as masturbating on a street corner. On each of these occasions, Mr. H, who had been using cocaine, was clinically manic. He had already been diagnosed with stroke disease and cognitive impairment, if not early dementia, due to it.

After each of these manic episodes, Mr. H would become profoundly depressed and need another 24 hours, if not more, of observation due to the depression alone. This is typical of the period after coming down from a cocaine or stimulant high, as all the neurotransmitters that elevate mood have now been washed away. This means that the vesicles at the terminal end of the nerve cell, normally holding the neurotransmitters that would be expelled into the synapse to stimulate the next nerve, are now empty. In 24 hours, an elated and sex-crazed person with mania will become depressed and suicidal with zero interest in anything sexual. Each time Mr. H went through this, his blood pressure soared, he suffered more small strokes, and his dementia progressed. Finally, one day Mr. H was found motionless in Central Park, his pants down and a hand on his penis. He was dead of a massive stroke.

## ALCOHOL AND DEMENTIA

Alcohol (ethanol), with its own sexual implications, is linked to dementia.

Ethyl alcohol has been a part of the human condition for so long that we actually have an enzyme, coded in our DNA, which specifically metabolizes it. This is the reason we can tolerate ethanol but not methanol (wood alcohol) or isopropyl (rubbing) alcohol. Nonetheless, desperate alcoholics are known to abuse methanol and isopropyl when ethanol is not readily available. The result of this practice is similar to exposing oneself to any other industrial solvent with all of their toxic effects.

The enzyme that allows us to tolerate ethanol is called alcohol dehydrogenase (there are 10 forms of it in our bodies). Younger men, in their 20s, contain about twice as much as women of similar age, which is why the former can tolerate more alcohol than the latter. As we age, the amount of the enzyme decreases, which is why less tolerance is part of growing older.

However, tolerance should be kept in the proper context. Alcohol is used, and abused, largely due to the nature of the delirium it causes. Generally speaking, there is a sense of well-being and a lowering of anxiety levels. For some, use of alcohol can be controlled, even when used regularly, socially, or when eating. For others, a single drink is the beginning of a cascade that must be curtailed or it will lead to the severe physical, mental, and social consequences that are identified as the disease called alcoholism.

While social stress, anxiety, mood disorders, and chronic mental illness have been associated with alcohol abuse, personal genetics predisposing one to alcoholism play an important role in the overall morbidity and mortality. A greatly abbreviated list of the consequences include suicide, homicide, domestic violence, liver disease, and a variety of brain abnormalities.

The most well-known results of drinking include a relaxation of social and sexual inhibitions. Nonetheless, acute alcohol intoxication or alcohol delirium is, for all intents and purposes, a form of mania.

But in addition to the delirium alcohol can cause, there is the relationship that it has to dementia. The direct destruction of brain tissue by chronic alcohol use is called alcohol dementia. And while there is some data to suggest that light alcohol consumption use may be preventative to the development of dementia, it has been estimated in one study that 10 percent of dementia in patients under the age of 64 is alcohol related.

In the medical community, the identification of alcohol dementia and the terminology used to describe it has been murky. Classic alcohol-related confusion, other than acute intoxication or withdrawal, is usually thought of as a part of Wernicke–Korsakoff syndrome. However, there are actually two separate problems. Wernicke–Korsakoff syndrome is a vitamin B1, or thiamine, deficiency caused by the poor nutritional intake, inadequate absorption, and improper cellular utilization of this vitamin. The earlier Wernicke stage is characterized by a staggering gait, eye movement abnormalities on one or both sides, and confusion (all three findings are present in one-third of cases) and is generally considered reversible.

The later Korsakoff psychosis is usually considered irreversible and believed by many to be alcohol dementia at that point. Some consider true alcohol dementia to be more of a direct result of the toxic effects of alcohol on the brain rather than a vitamin deficiency. However, in practice the two are often difficult to separate.

This is a peculiar dementia. It may begin as early as 30 years old or as late as 80, and may involve a variety of cognitive dysfunctions, including memory loss. What most cases seem to have in common is the easily missed confabulation, a sort of elaborate fibbing or story-telling around the memory loss and confusion. Only when pinning the patient down on the details can an examiner begin to decipher just how much confusion is present. It's a lesson I learned from Leo.

I first met Leo at a skilled nursing facility where I was consulting. As I was walking in, he and an attractive woman were walking out, and I held the door for them. They said "thank you" and I thought nothing of it. As I went about my business, the word started to circulate that a man named Leo was missing. "Who is Leo?" I asked a nurse. When she described him—a man in his late 50s, handsome, well-dressed, and well-spoken—I realized I had just abetted in the getaway and told her what had transpired. I suspected that he couldn't have gotten far, and indeed, the staff found him in the parking lot, behind the wheel of a car and backing out. The woman he was with was asked to take the car and leave. Leo was escorted back to his appointment—with me.

It turned out that Leo was from a well-to-do-family. Though there was a certain polish to his personality, he was also a raging alcoholic, had been so for years, and was formally diagnosed with alcohol dementia. Despite his confusion, he was able to slide past considerable barriers before being identified as someone who was very confused. Even his fiduciary, who oversaw the amount of money given to him and who I met that day, was amazed at how normal Leo could seem. The trustee told me, "His family demanded that a fiduciary be assigned to him and that he be given a substantial allowance each month and be allowed some freedom to come and go from the facility. They don't realize how confused he is now. But the ladies, they know exactly what is going on and will take him for all they can get. Some of them are prostitutes and some of them come from only God knows where. Still, he has a way of finding them."

I spent quite a bit of time with Leo that day. Despite being very confused and psychotic, he went on and on in a very sophisticated and fluent matter as if nothing at all was wrong with him. According to him, he was a professor of higher mathematics at the University of Washington and just back from a sabbatical in Jakarta. Trying to change the subject frequently, he queried me about what I knew about the island of Java and where Jakarta was located.

In a not so subtle way, Leo derided me for my lack of Indonesian travel experience, especially my being unaware of the vast pool of beauty to be found in nearby Papua, New Guinea. I thanked him for adding to my database, telling him I had only been aware of Kuru there, a rapidly fatal dementia related to mad cow disease, which is transmitted via cannibalism. With that, he excused himself to "get back to his girlfriend."

This time he was prevented from exiting the premises. As the director of nursing reminded him, his girlfriend was one of many who had been ordered to stay away from him and the facility. Enraged, Leo stormed off to his room.

A week later, Leo attempted to hire an attorney to contest the limitations being set on him. Fortunately, his psychosis was not as attractive to the lawyer as it was to his lovers. Yet, not to be deterred, Leo soon went missing again not long after receiving a new installment of cash. One week later he was found nude and beaten in a local park.

At that point Adult Protective Services finally got involved and, superseding the naïve desires of his family, a formal guardianship was assigned to him. That this hadn't happened earlier almost got Leo killed.

Alcohol is one substance linked to dementia. There is another substance that is also linked to dementia and it too has sexual implications. We ingest it every day. And while not everyone drinks, everyone eats.

## SUGAR AND DEMENTIA

It is well known that refined sugar, present in so many food items beyond candy and soda, is closely linked to type-2 diabetes. It is also important to note that an immune response—an inflammation—occurs whenever sugar is eaten, thereby setting the stage for the development of atherosclerosis, the dangerous fatty plaques lining arteries.

Atherosclerosis and diabetes are clearly associated with one another, as well as with a number of serious medical conditions, including strokes and heart attacks. It's not a leap, therefore, to connect the overconsumption of refined sugars to the development of dementia. While this ability to process refined sugar varies from person to person according to our genetics, it has been well established on a societal level that the amount of sugar consumed nationwide is a serious health concern.

*I believe that there is no one regularly ingested substance more closely associated with dementia than refined sugar.*

Until recently, I would have said that this was more the case with vascular dementia than the other causes due to the link between diabetes and strokes. However, new evidence suggests that even Alzheimer's disease may be associated with a diabetic condition existing within the cells of the brain. This revelation has led to new research where inhaled insulin is being studied for the treatment of Alzheimer's disease.

So, how does sugar consumption itself affect sexuality? Low blood sugar, possibly as the result of an insulin reaction from an injection, or even our own insulin (this is known as reactive hypoglycemia), will usually bring about a depressed and irritable mood. Whether or not one suffers from dementia, this situation is not conducive to sexual desire or activity. However, someone with dementia cannot say or understand what is happening within his or her body. The onus is on the caregiver to do a full assessment in all cases of mental status changes in those with dementia, because there are many various mental state changes associated with low or high sugar levels. This is especially true in dementia patients, as their brains are so vulnerable. Annabelle showed me how sugar delirium can drive sexual behavior.

Annabelle was an 85-year-old woman with mild dementia who was brought to the emergency department on Mother's Day. She was described as a kind and soft-spoken person who carried a Bible with her everywhere she went. Annabelle was also a diabetic.

Her family knew something was wrong when Annabelle rose out of the church pew and into the aisle, chanting and hollering to the music. "At first it was a little funny," her son told me. "But then the words that I never thought were inside that woman came out. We covered the ears of the kids and hauled her out of there!"

The words hadn't stopped at the doors of the ER. Annabelle was loud, feeling good, and ready to have sex with just about anybody there. We had to tie her down and give her an injection of a tranquilizer just to draw blood. That test revealed a blood sugar level of over 1,000. A normal reading is around 100.

Annabelle was admitted to the hospital and treated for high blood sugar–related delirium and diabetic ketoacidosis, a related metabolic condition. When I passed by her room the next day, Annabelle greeted me. She dropped her reading glasses—she had been reading her Bible—and was as sweet as could be.

***Do's and Don'ts on Substances, Drugs, and Sexual Behavior***

- Do consider a substance or drug at the root of a new sexual behavior
- Do consider a toxicology screen
- Do evaluate the diet with a nutritionist
- Do have the doctor review all medications
- Don't assume it's just the person
- Don't assume it's just the dementia

## CAUSE AND EFFECT

There are many specific situations where mental status changes occur due to either a metabolic change or the ingestion of a drug or a substance. There are many more in addition to the ones mentioned in this chapter. That is why it is imperative that caregivers continually monitor the medical status, medications, and nutrition of dementia patients. All of these factors can be the basis for unexpected sexual behavior. Recognizing them is the first step to treating sexual issues.

CHAPTER NINE

# Treating the Symptoms

Dementia treatment requires a thorough understanding of what is, or isn't, normal, acceptable, and safe. This knowledge reaches well beyond individual psychology and neurochemistry. Regulations, policies, relationships, and family values also become a part of a complex situation that differs in every case.

In a long-term care or medical facility, when a sexual behavior is deemed to be problematic, it must be fully assessed and the details documented. A detailed narrative, usually by a nurse, a social worker, or both, is written. The facility will then determine, based upon regulatory pressure, treatment outcome, and other factors, whether or not it can continue to keep the patient as a resident without some sort of hospital intervention.

The home situation vis-à-vis sexual behavior is different. There is no protocol, policy, or procedure for documentation. Not infrequently, a spouse will put up with the behavior for a long time due to personal commitment and lack of any knowledge of either how to deal with such a matter or the governing regulations other than domestic violence laws. Identification of a problem and reporting it are major obstacles one must contend with in the home situation.

Regardless of the situation, safety for all of those involved is always the number one priority when it comes to intervention and treatment of any behavior, sexual or not. This must be accomplished quickly and decisively through whatever means available.

Once safety for all involved is achieved, a treatment can begin. The emphasis on the handling of sexual problems related to dementia should generally focus on the following, in order: medical, environmental, behavioral, and then pharmacological (medication) approaches. Each of these may be divided into a passive, or preventive, approach as well as an active one. A passive or preventative method will always be the starting place. For example, keeping a living situation or routine or medication that is working well is always preferred over intervening and making changes when sexual symptoms arise.

Dementia is dynamic; it always progresses slowly with occasional sudden bumps. Reactions of family, friends, and caregivers who don't expect the sexual behaviors, much less know how to cope with them, can range from denial to disgust. The experienced care professional will learn to recognize when the passive approach has failed and determine when medical, environmental, behavioral, or pharmacologic treatment is necessary. He or she will also realize that various elements of treatment will often need to be utilized simultaneously.

***Dealing with Dementia and Behaviors***

It's crucial to remember the following:

- Neither staff nor family should have to tolerate behaviors that make them uncomfortable.
- Don't fight. Leave the situation and seek help from family, supervisors, an emergency room, or authorities.
- If you are a professional caregiver, read the company policy on workplace safety.
- Once you are safe and away, use the reported behaviors constructively to help the person involved.

## THE GOLDEN RULE

The standard initial treatment—the Golden Rule—for all mental status concerns, especially in the elderly, is to first address what treatable medical issues could be causing the symptoms. Sometimes obvious yet forgotten medical concerns may be at the root of agitation, depression, or anxiety. These might include a bladder full of urine in a man with an enlarged prostate, constipation, or arthritic pain. It is well known that delirium and side effects to medications may play a role in sexual symptoms. It is also known that those with dementia are especially vulnerable to such side effects due to the sensitivity of their brains. Given these circumstances, it makes sense that any new behavioral concern in a dementia patient deserves a complete medical evaluation. That includes a physical examination, along with laboratory and radiographic studies to rule out infection or metabolic instability, such as a urinary tract infection or high blood sugar. Medication needs to be reviewed, especially if something new has been started. Ralph's case was a textbook example.

An 80-year-old man with mild dementia and chronic bronchitis from smoking, Ralph developed flu-like symptoms not long after a visit from his children and grandchildren, most of whom had just gotten over bad winter colds. He was placed on antibiotics by his primary doctor, who was concerned about Ralph's mucus-producing cough. Things went from bad to worse quickly. Jan, his wife, called 911 in the middle of the night after finding Ralph wandering around the house with his clothes off.

In the ER Ralph was more confused and sexually inappropriate with the nurses. I met Ralph and Jan the next day on the medical floor. Ralph had been diagnosed with delirium due to pneumonia and an exacerbation of his chronic obstructive pulmonary disease (COPD) and placed on IV antibiotics and Prednisone, a steroid. (Steroids are often given in cases of exacerbated COPD, especially with pneumonia, because they are anti-inflammatory and act quickly.) He had to be restrained to keep his hands off the nurses, so we started IV antipsychotics as well. "This is so embarrassing," Jan said. "He's never done anything like this before."

To my surprise, a day later he was worse. We were unable to wean him out of restraints due to his extreme agitation accompanied by vulgarities and provocative sexual threats. He was loud, excited, and elated. In short, he was manic. "This is terrible," Jan exclaimed. "He's worse. Do something now, please!"

The internist and I sat in the nurse's station and brainstormed. I think we both said "the Prednisone" at the same time. We discussed the options with Jane. We could begin to lower the Prednisone more quickly than usual, but his respiratory condition could worsen. Or we could sedate him. In either case, he could end up on a ventilator and in the ICU. The other option was to ride out the mania, but his being restrained was dangerous, too. Physical restraint can cause overexertion involving increased blood pressure and pulse and put stress on the heart and brain. Death can even result. Using meds as fast as possible to get rid of the physical restraint is always preferred.

Jan, after being advised of the choices, told us, "I understand I have to make a choice. I cannot stand to see this man, who showed such dignity throughout our marriage, in this condition. But no ICU; that is not an option he would want. Not with the dementia, not with his age. He's lived a long life. Let's see what happens here on this floor only. It's in God's hands."

We agreed on a compromise, which was to lower the Prednisone slowly and add a little sedation. Sadly, 24 hours later, Ralph died of respiratory failure.

### *Medical Management Options for Treating Sexual Behaviors*

**The Passive Approach**

- Routine physical examination
- One doctor prescribing medications
- Healthy living with emphasis on activity, exercise, and nutrition

**The Active Approach**

- Any mental status change in a dementia patient is viewed as delirium until proven otherwise
- A medical history and examination should be obtained
- A review of current medications and recent changes should be performed
- Appropriate laboratory studies may be needed to assess for infection, intoxication, or metabolic disturbance

## THE FOUR PASSIVE STEPS IN BEHAVIORAL MANAGEMENT OF SEXUAL BEHAVIORS

### *The First Passive Step: Maintenance of the Living Environment*

For couples, it is important to recognize and understand that passive action requires recognizing and understanding the aspects of day-to-day living, which reflect intimacy. Sex or romance is commonly tied to *familiarity and routine, which are the solid foundation of dementia care*. Critical to any memory care unit, but silently present in all home situations as well, these are often the pillars that crack at the moment the first major dementia-related behavioral event occurs. This event is often associated with a cognitive decline, which can be measured.

For example, one of the three popular cognitive rating scales can be used. They are the Mini Mental Status Examination (MMSE), the St. Louis University Mental Status examination (SLUMS) or the Montreal Cognitive Assessment test (MoCA). There is an additional assessment known as Saint Andrews Sexual Behavior Assessment (SASBA): it is one of the few measurement tools available for assessing the type and severity of sexual behaviors, but it is seldom used in the United States. I believe the reason is that there has never been an objective reason to quantify its use in a study.

Each cognitive scale rates the patient's cognitive abilities on a scale of 0 to 30. Roughly, a score in the 20s is consistent with early dementia, the teens with moderate disease, and less than 10 with advanced disease.

A sudden change in the daily familiarity or routine by virtue of just about anything—an illness, a vacation, a move to a new residence—can drop the score of someone with dementia by five points or more overnight. I call this *environmental regression*. One common misconception of this phenomenon is that the environmental change caused the dementia. The reality is that the dementia was already there, lingering, unnoticed or denied, held in check until there is an imbalance and life begins to tumble.

Sexuality, familiarity, and routine join to form the basis of living for many of us. As though lacking in oxygen, the sexual spark will not burn a flame for long without the familiarity and routine that help to feed love, the ultimate fuel in any relationship. This is why lust fades as familiarity and routine develop. From there, one either falls in love, moves into a dysfunctional relationship, or moves on.

Now imagine being old and in love and romantic with your spouse of 59 years. Perhaps without regular sexual activity, but with important things like kisses, rubs, and touches, you go about each day feeling connected, whole, and content. And then suddenly, she or he—that person, that presence—disappears emotionally. What could be more painful than that first heartbreak at 16? This could. And for those with dementia, hanging onto reality by a thread, this is beyond heartbreak; it is disastrous. You can count on trouble from there on in.

I met Peggy and Mel years ago. They had been married nearly 60 years and were very much in love. Life was good, despite the fact that they each suffered with some mild dementia. Their daughter lived across the street and looked in on them regularly, and they received four hours of home care each day. Then, while weeding the lawn one spring, Mel slipped, hit the ground, and broke his hip.

He underwent surgery and moved to a nursing home for rehab for a month after that. He gradually became stronger physically, but his confusion rapidly grew worse. Peggy fell apart during his absence. The daughter tried as much as possible to keep her going with the same routine but she sank deeper and deeper into confusion. By week three, despite routine visits together, Peggy and Mel hardly recognized one another. The daughter was devastated and perplexed until I explained to her the power of the love and familiarity they had with one another. Eventually, Peggy and Mel were reunited in an assisted-living facility, but life was never the same. They seemed to barely know one another. It was as though the candle had burned out.

The case of Peggy and Mel is instructive on the power of romantic routine and familiarity. Sadly, in so many cases nothing can be done.

Whether you are a caregiver in the home or in a long-term care facility, learning to confront sexual behaviors is a challenge. At home, either spouse may quickly become a victim if steps are not taken to confront the behavior. In long-term care, patients of either sex might exhibit behaviors, but the fact is that the workforce greatly tilts toward women, many of whom are young and inexperienced. This combination makes them particularly vulnerable to sexual behaviors. One obvious difference between home and long-term care is that, in the case of the spouse or partner, sexual behavior between the patient and caregiver may have occurred in the past and may still be happening. In contrast, caregivers in long-term facilities are never to engage in, or to encourage, sexual activity with a patient.

### *The Second Passive Step: Identifying Discomfort*

No care provider, spouse, or professional should tolerate being in a sexually uncomfortable situation. This is, at times, hard to do, especially without experience, as one often feels sympathy for a confused patient. The result is allowance for more inappropriate comments and gestures and possibly even sex acts in the case of the spouse or partner who would otherwise rather not participate. Other than sympathy, someone might feel they will further exacerbate or inflame the situation or that things might escalate into anger or danger.

Sympathy at the expense of one's comfort and integrity is false sympathy. That one might further diminish a dementia patient's life by setting limits on sexual behavior is false. That things might further escalate if the desired sexual behavior is not allowed is also false; in fact, the reverse is true. This requires constant self-examination on the part of the caregiver and a commitment to resolving the problem. That's exactly what Milo and Kay discovered.

Kay put up with Milo's demands for most of their marriage. When he became demented, the trend continued because Kay never learned to set limits on him. He would continue to pursue her sexually, with little resistance, although Kay was very uncomfortable with the situation. Finally their three daughters made an intervention whereby one of them moved in with Milo and Kay and insisted on separate sleeping quarters for each parent. This was met with considerable anger from Milo until it was made clear that his next option was a nursing home. Things calmed down considerably after that.

### *The Third Passive Step: Avoiding Provocation*

Avoiding provocation involves insight on the part of the spouse, partner, or caregiver because that person's very presence might provoke sexual behavior on the part of the patient. This is especially true if the person is the opposite sex.

A confused patient senses the way a person looks, smells, and walks the same way anyone else does. These other senses actually may be heightened. Add that to less ability to contain the reactive feelings and the situation is ripe for sexual behaviors.

The content of conversation should be neutral and kept away from anything provocative. For instance, a spouse talking about romance on the beach 40 years ago may be looking for sexual behavior. A caregiver in a nursing home sharing personal information may have an unexpected surprise in store. Taylor found this out the hard way.

A cute, 22-year-old female nursing assistant in a memory care assisted living facility, with two babies at home being cared for by her mother, an Army husband currently deployed to Afghanistan, and working toward a nursing degree part-time, Taylor was under a great deal of stress. Nonetheless, she thought she found an outlet for her stress with 76-year-old Mr. Colgate, who was quite lonely as well. They often sat on his bed and talked, sharing stories about their personal lives, including romance. On occasion she would hug him, and she once kissed him on the cheek.

And then came the day that would change everything. While sitting next to Mr. Colgate on the bed, charting the vital signs in her book, his hand slowly landed on her breast. Taylor jumped up, startling Mr. Colgate, who still wore a pleasant and loving smile. Red-faced, she ran from the room and her job.

I heard this story from Taylor, an RN on our unit, 10 years later. She hadn't considered how her close relationship to Mr. Colgate was associated with the absence of her father and her own inappropriately flirtatious grandfather. With just a touch, she told me, she suddenly became aware of both. She had needed that closeness with an older man, and yet this conflicted with her deep feelings of resentment over Mr. Colgate's abuse. She had worked through this over the years to the point that she was able to understand it and talk about it.

This is a reminder that working with dementia patients is, in some ways, like working with a tabula rasa, a blank slate that is available for us caregivers to work through our own inner issues. It would behoove any of us to develop insight into such issues in order to give the best care possible to our patients.

### *The Fourth Passive Step: Creating Barriers*

Barriers are a matter of limiting the likelihood of an event and providing for safety. This is similar to environmental concerns, but with more of an immediate behavioral management focus rather than a longer term environmental solution. Patients who have a known history of sexual issues should be placed with roommates that are less vulnerable. A presence of particular staff, such as a male nurse, may be a deterrent. Moving a staff member who is the object of desire away from that particular patient only makes sense. A female caregiver should not find herself deep inside the room with a confused man she does not know well who is guarding the door.

During a bath or caregiving, especially peri care—attention of the perineal area, such as washing the genitals—anticipate events. This is a time to be mindful of potential groping. Several staff may be required to assure that all involved are comfortable with the procedure.

Despite passive measures, oftentimes behaviors will emerge, regardless of what measures have been taken, and one must be prepared to take active steps while the passive steps remain in place.

## THE FOUR ACTIVE STEPS IN BEHAVIORAL MANAGEMENT OF SEXUAL BEHAVIORS

Many times a passive behavioral approach is simply not enough. Family pressures, as well as safety concerns, join with the behaviors of the patients to create a perfect storm that must be dealt with swiftly. Moving someone to his or her room, separation of patients, support from other caregivers, and even calling 911, if necessary, may all be steps needed to provide safety, control of the situation, and retreat of an angry or aggressive family. Certainly, in long-term care, documentation of the event and evaluation of those involved, including a trip to the hospital for either medical or psychiatric care, also may be required to ensure complete satisfaction to all involved.

For example, Mickey and Don, each with dementia, had become quite fond of one another at the assisted living. They made it clear they were in love and wanted to have sex. Each believed that the other was a spouse, and they were becoming more passionate about one another by the minute. Complicating (or simplifying, depending on one's outlook) matters was that the real spouse and family of each would visit routinely. The staff arranged a meeting where they all were made aware of the romance. They did not approve of it in the least. Everyone quickly agreed that Mickey and Don would be repositioned to opposite ends of the building as a preventative measure. They did run into one another now and then, but the fire was gone.

### *The First Active Step: Manipulating the Environment*

Most often there is time to plan an act in a manner that will prevent last-minute anxieties or distress. Keeping a couple together is always preferable, but at times some imaginative action goes a long way to remedy the situation.

Andy, 78, and James, 80, were a gay couple who lived in an assisted living center. They had been together for more than 40 years. James had dementia and Andy was very reliant upon his partner. One day I received a call from a nurse who explained the situation further: "Andy is just getting the daylights beaten out of him by James. Every time we try and separate them, they both go through the roof. We don't know what to do. Help!"

I met with them a day later. Andy was indeed very dependent on James and found it difficult to take a position on his injuries, which amounted to scratches and bruising on his arms. "We're fine in the morning," he began. "Then the afternoon comes and he needs a kiss and a hug, and before you know it I'm having an affair with Mr. Kim next door. By dinnertime it starts to get physical, and I don't mean having sex!" I asked Andy why he put up with it so long. He started to cry. "I don't know what I'd do without him. He needs me, and obviously I need him."

James was significantly confused and no doubt sundowning each afternoon. While Andy was more vocal about a separation, it would probably be James who would deteriorate the most. It could mean the end for them living together. I reviewed James's medications and considered something to help take the edge off his afternoons but his guardian was against any psychiatric medications.

I met with the staff. We reckoned that training Andy to take a more aggressive position would only inflame James more—if Andy was even able to do that. Our options were limited: no meds, plus they couldn't have somebody in the room all afternoon and night. It seemed that some sort of strategic separation was going to be necessary to maintain enough of the familiarity and routine of the relationship in the morning for James and yet protect Andy in the afternoon. About then it occurred to me to ask, "What is Andy even doing in assisted-living all day anyway? He's a high-functioning intact guy." At that point, the staff realized how everyone had been drawn into Andy's dependency, seeing him as almost as incapable as James.

The next few months were rocky, as there was resistance to our plan, which was to keep them together while providing for the disparate needs of each partner. Happily, the plan worked. Eventually, Andy was able to obtain part-time work in an art store in the afternoon, while James was engaged in therapeutic activities geared toward those with early to moderate dementia. By suppertime the two were ready to reunite, generally without incident. James was tired in the evening due to the activities and went to bed earlier. Andy did seem a little more assertive, too. With that came a new level of responsibility and caregiver attitude toward James that had not been present before. It was a good nonmedication solution that actually improved the conditions of the patients.

But inevitably there are times when a very aggressive and active approach needs to be taken when it comes to the environment and sexual behaviors. Most commonly this involves a patient, often a man, who is repeatedly predatory with patients or staff or both. Such patients will have had multiple unsuccessful attempts of stabilization from all possible therapeutic avenues, including medication and behavioral strategies. Placement or environmental change is often the only solution. Such patients are notoriously difficult because they cannot live alone, the family cannot manage them, and few facilities are going to be interested in someone with such a symbolic red flag who already may be secluded or on one-to-one observation. Such was the case of Ernie, an 87-year-old man with moderate dementia.

The former commissioner of a major West Coast port, Ernie was well-known throughout the neighborhood. His family had done a good job of working with the community in an effort to raise awareness of Alzheimer's disease. Their openness about Ernie's illness was admirable but reached its limits with the onset of sexual behaviors. Ernie had already been at several memory care facilities—he was asked to leave because of fondling patients and staff—when I met him on our inpatient unit.

His wife and two daughters broke down on our first meeting together. "This is so not my husband," Clarice, his wife, said. "He was always such a gentle and respectful man and now, this. Who's going to want him? Sedate him if you have to. I just want him somewhere that he can last." I knew what she meant, not that she wanted him hidden, but that he deserved some quality of life somewhere, and all the moving around was not giving him anything like that. The social workers and I knew this was going to be a challenge. We managed to stabilize Ernie with medication and minimal sedation, but knew there was no guarantee he'd stay stable and not require more without the right environment. There were a couple of adult family homes that only took men, but they were full. Eventually we convinced a small adult family home looking for challenging patients that he would be just right for them.

In the end it was his cooperative and understanding family, working with the new facility, that was the strength of this case. The caregivers in the small adult family home knew they would have full support of the family to create a protective environment that was conducive to Ernie regaining his life without isolating him from others. The family was also willing to allow for sedation, and even end-of-life care, if it meant a stable and lasting living situation for him.

This case demonstrates how economy and balance of attributes so commonly a concern of families—sedation, activity level, and freedom—will change through the course of a dementia, particularly when sexual behaviors are involved.

A note about end-of-life care: At times, no matter what is done, the choices are stark. Either the patient has behaviors or he is sedated. The latter is generally preferred, assuming the family agrees; otherwise placement will be impossible. Comfort care, quietly done behind the scenes, is common, but formal hospice care still requires more medical diagnoses so that insurers, including Medicare, will pay. In 2012, only 12.8 percent of Americans in hospice care had a primary diagnosis of dementia, according to statistics from the National Hospice and Palliative Care Organization. The number is up from 7 percent in 2001, but it is still a small proportion given the country's galloping rates of dementia.

### *The Second Active Step: Redirection*

Redirection is a well-known technique in behavioral management of dementia patients. It involves psychologically or physically redirecting a thought or activity to something or someplace more appropriate. Examples include taking someone masturbating in public to their room, steering a conversation that is getting sexually heated to one less so, redirecting two confused patients about to kiss to an activity group, or a spouse taking her husband out for a walk rather than continue to avoid his advances in the house.

Redirection is generally considered best if combined with validation to some degree, so as not to make the patient feel bad. However, this should be balanced with limit setting and making sure that the inappropriateness of the behavior is discussed. Limitations of this approach include the very nature of dementia and the likelihood of having to repeat this strategy more than once. Here's an example.

Ken rapidly approached Wanda, a nurse on our inpatient service. She backed up, with a smile, into a corner, holding a cup of water in one hand and a cup of another patient's medications in the other. Ken, smiling, was staring at her breasts. He slowed his approach but seemed to be headed toward something inappropriate. Wanda stayed calm and started a conversation to redirect him: "Kenny, I know you like to smile and talk with me, but the group is starting right now in the other room and you are late." Ken looked up for the room where he was expected as Wanda slid out of the corner and moved into an area where there was a group of staff and other patients. Ken still smiled at Wanda but became so caught up in the change of plans that he was redirected to another line of thinking. Best of all, he remained on good terms with Wanda.

### *The Third Active Step: Limit Setting*

There are times when, no matter what caregivers do, the behavior just keeps happening. This may include exposing oneself, making inappropriate comments, or even physical touching. In most cases, the action will create an uncomfortable situation that must be addressed. Oftentimes, redirection is simply not enough, and limits or boundaries must be set.

The first part of this step is to identify what the limits are and how much should be allowed. This might be based upon your discomfort or that of others, safety issues, specific policies, and at times just plain common sense.

Secondly, after consultation with a supervisor if need be, firm but respectful communication of these limits and boundaries needs to be made. This may take the form of a specific action, place, or time. It should be done in a straightforward and serious way. Remember that blame is not the goal; stopping the behavior is. If there are consequences, they should be laid out as well. All should be carefully thought out beforehand in order to ensure appropriateness and certainty of the consequences. Care planning, or a family meeting, can be helpful for this. In fact, it is often preferable to have a group or team as a part of the limit setting, as this will underscore the resolve and seriousness. It will also prevent any attempt of the patient to leave as a defense against this technique.

### *The Fourth Active Step: Care Planning*

Because each individual is different, with varying motives, strengths, and weaknesses, it is always helpful to carefully plan an approach to recurrent problematic sexual behaviors. In the case of a facility, this should be done with a treatment team. At home, other family, the physician, or an in-home care assistant should be recruited into service. From there, differences should be sorted out in order to approach the problem as a unified front. Any division or inconsistency will only weaken the plan and set it up to fail.

The overall plan of care that addresses the problem should be discussed thoroughly with safety and quality of life at the core. Policies and regulations may need to be revisited, staff may need training, and families may need to make major adjustments. Regardless, all involved must make a commitment that the cycle of the behavior will end, no matter what the cost. Otherwise, one must assume either the behavior does not warrant stopping or that there must be some other reason it would be allowed to continue.

***Behavioral Approaches for Treating Sexual Behaviors***

All these approaches are to be conducted simultaneously:

**Passive**

1. Environmental maintenance
2. Identifying discomfort
3. Avoiding provocation
4. Creating barriers

**Active**

1. Environmental manipulation
2. Redirection
3. Limit setting
4. Care planning

## THE PHARMACOLOGIC MANAGEMENT OF SEXUAL BEHAVIORS

If, after delirium has been ruled out and environmental and behavioral approaches have been carefully thought out and instituted, sexual behaviors are still ongoing, the next line of treatment is medication.

When doing anything with a drug to achieve some goal, it is helpful to keep in mind that the same beneficial effect that a drug may give in one situation might be an unwanted side effect in another situation. This may be the case with sexual side effects, too (see chapter 8). On a psychological level for example, a dementia medication may allow someone the wherewithal to be sexual yet it may be inappropriate at times. Stopping such a medication may lead to sinking into more confusion and exhibiting less problematic behaviors, yet the patient will no longer be a sexual individual. A balance must be considered. Another situation is on a more biological level, as with the antidepressants. Increasing a mood usually enhances sexuality, but overmedicate and a manic situation might be struck where too much sexuality occurs. Complicating matters further, a major side effect of some antidepressants—for other reasons—is one of lack of sexual desire or function.

The basic choices are:

- Antidementia medication
- Antidepressant medication
- Mood stabilizers
- Antianxiety medication
- Antipsychotic medication
- Hormonal therapy

It should be noted that making a decision to use any medication is serious. The elderly are more sensitive to medications, not to mention the likelihood that the person already takes several drugs. Every attempt should be made to limit the amount and types of medications used. One is the preferred number. There should also be a plan in place to eventually reduce and discontinue the medication, unless this is a long-term regimen such as antidementia drugs or hormonal therapy.

## DEMENTIA MEDICATION: WHEN IS THE RIGHT TIME TO STOP?

Dementia is regarded as a condition that requires long-term treatment, but there are a couple of reasons to stop earlier:

1. There comes a time where the dementia is so far progressed that there seems to be no reason to keep the patient on such a medication. At that point, it's time to cut down a lot of other meds (e.g., cholesterol drugs) as well.
2. When the behaviors are really bad and hard to treat, the determination should be made whether cognitive ability is fueling the situation. Sometimes, by lowering the cognitive ability (assuming stopping the drug will make any difference at all, which more often than not it doesn't), the behaviors improve.

Maddie, who developed an Alzheimer's-type of dementia at 65, illustrates the point. The disease was slow to progress and had been diagnosed early. She and her husband, Rick, studied the benefits of antidementia drugs and realized treatment was likely to buy quality time for them, maybe even three years or more. Her outpatient neurologist, Dr. T—a friend of mine—started her on the Exelon patch (rivastigmine).

Very likely due to this medication, the couple was able to enjoy a fairly normal life over the next five years. Though Rick saw the gradual deterioration, he compensated by taking over more and more of the household duties. They remained very much in love and sexually active through it all. Rick would tell me later that this was the most precious time of their entire 40 years together, and he partially thanked the Exelon patch for that.

Eventually a point came where things became less manageable. Maddie was getting paranoid and excessively flirtatious in public. She was hospitalized with us for a violent episode related to her conviction that Rick was having an affair. Rick and I discussed all the options. He strongly felt that her disease had progressed "to the point where she is struggling, like someone drowning. I think if she goes under, she'll feel better and be in a better place."

I agreed with him, and as a part of the treatment we agreed to stop the patch. I told him there was a chance it would make no difference at all, or she might crash cognitively and never recognize him again, yet retain or even experience more aggression and psychosis. He knew the score.

A week later, Maddie was in another world. She was more confused and unaware of who Rick was, but, because of that, she was no longer paranoid or distressed. It was hard for him to see her go so fast, yet he was grateful for the new place she found herself.

## BEING IN THE MOOD: THE ANTIDEPRESSANTS

The antidepressants are a class of medication that plays a dual role when it comes to sexual behaviors in dementia patients. All the drugs, both old and new, are capable of driving a dementia patient into a state of mania. This is due to the sensitivity of the dementia patient's brain to shifts in the neurotransmitter milieu. Mania comes with a variety of symptoms and hypersexuality is commonly one of them. Dotty's case is a good example.

I first met Dotty at an assisted-living center where she had presented with isolative behavior, poor appetite, and anxiety. While she had a known case of Alzheimer's disease, depression had clearly taken the primary spot on her problem list. Her primary care doctor had done a great job of obtaining a history from the family. It revealed a somewhat dependent personality that they felt was at play in her sad reaction to the change to assisted living a year after her spouse had passed. The physical examination was unrevealing, as were the basic lab findings. (These were a CBC, which includes a white blood and red blood cell count; a BMP or basic metabolic panel, with information about the basic electrolytes sodium and potassium, plus kidney function and blood sugar; and a urinalysis to rule out a urinary tract infection.)

The doctor then ordered Remeron (mirtazapine), an antidepressant often given to improve appetite. This medicine was soon stopped due to some side effects that Dotty was reporting, such as dizziness, headache, and nausea. Coincidentally, this particular family was somewhat overly sensitive and concerned about their "dependent" mother. This only added to the pressure for the doctor to stop the medication. Then he tried Celexa (citalopram), a great middle-of-the-road serotonin reuptake inhibitor, but Dotty again cited the vague side effects that prompted another medication discontinuation.

By the time I entered the picture as the psychiatric consultant, the family was distressed and somewhat demanding. They had decided that Prozac (fluoxetine)—something half of them had taken in the past or was currently on—was the way to go. Okay, I thought, another SSRI, generally okay in younger people, very long half-life (it takes forever to get out of the system once stopped), very activating with potential anxiety and jitteriness, and not great for appetite. Do they really want to do this?

Given the recent issues with this family (I thought the patient would have done fine on the other medications if they'd stayed out of it), I saw a real problem brewing. Dotty could do great. However, we could be putting her on a drug with side effects that would take a long time to get out of her system. I explained my concerns to the family but they had already decided: Prozac was the right drug for their mother.

Dotty tolerated the Prozac and actually began to improve within the first week. She was more social and active as well as eating better. "See Doc?" her son joked, "if you need any help in the future just let me know." Two weeks later she was laughing and elated. The family couldn't have been more pleased. She was no longer calling them in the middle of the night. They could finally sleep. The trouble was, Dotty wasn't sleeping well, and I was worried.

About three weeks after starting the Prozac, Dotty began going after men sexually. It started with talk and flirtation. At first, this one or that one was so handsome, but then it was more explicit, as she related what she would like to do with them. Her advances soon became predatory. Something had to be done.

I met with the no longer happy family. I told them the behavior was likely a manic episode caused by the Prozac, and the drug would have to be stopped. And worse, it would take two weeks for Dotty to calm down due to the long half-life of the drug. The facility said they couldn't safely care for her or the other residents without some tranquilization. The family was against that. There were two other options: either have a family member sit with her 24/7 at the facility (they couldn't afford one-to-one observation) or take her home. At the time, our hospital unit was full, with a waiting list. For two full weeks a family member was there. Eventually Dotty retreated back into her depression. We started over, this time my way, including a low dose of duloxetine (Cymbalta), which helped manage her anxiety as well as pain issues that had been overlooked. A swallow evaluation adjusted her diet to one more appropriate to her swallowing ability. Most importantly, we got her engaged in some creative arts and social activities to which she took a liking. She felt much better within a month.

Fortunately, mania, even in dementia patients, is not the most common outcome in the process of treating depression. More likely, sexuality, which was previously quelled by the negative mood, will improve to a normal level. Furthermore, and very much contrasting with the specter of mania in those who are vulnerable, such as dementia or bipolar patients, a well-known side effect of many antidepressants is a negative sexual one. This generally ranges from a loss of libido to a loss of orgasm, the latter especially in women. The basis is serotonin.

It turns out that, while this important brain chemical is critical to elevating our mood, it actually is inhibitory to our libido. As one might imagine, it is the antidepressants that rely most upon serotonin manipulation that have the most problem with this side effect. It's no surprise then, that those on SSRIs are particularly affected. On the other hand, those antidepressants with no serotonin effect tend to have limited or no sexual side effects.

***The Antidepressant/Serotonin Connection***

SSRIs, antidepressants with exclusive serotonin effect:
  Celexa, Paxil, Prozac, Zoloft
SRIs, antidepressants with mixed serotonin effect:
  Cymbalta, Effexor
Antidepressants with no serotonin effect:
  Remeron, Wellbutrin

*(continued)*

***The Antidepressant/Serotonin Connection (continued)***

When it comes to sexual behaviors in dementia patients, a dilemma exists with antidepressants. There is the risk of mania on the one hand and negative effects on sexuality on the other. In order to further portray this, let's take a look at the treatment disparities when considering the antidepressants in the face of inappropriate sexual behavior in a dementia patient.

I say find any antidepressant a patient might be on and stop it. This strategy comes from experience. The down side of this strategy is that the antidepressant might have had nothing to do with the behaviors, while the risk of a deeper depression lingers. Nonetheless, I believe that the risk of an irreversible depression—and even death—is outweighed by a simple medication maneuver that will often solve the problem. I am particularly confident in this approach if the antidepressant is new or starting it has coincided with the inception of the sexual behavior. On the other hand, someone historically stabilized from a severe and dangerous depression with the antidepressant in question, which, time-wise, has little to do with the sexual behavior, is less likely to be a good candidate for having it stopped.

Other clinicians take a different approach. They may also stop the antidepressant but with the intention to replace it with another, an SSRI antidepressant, with the hope that the sexual inhibitory side effects will win the day. If the patient is on nothing, they will start an SSRI anew. If the patient is already on an SSRI, they may increase it. The risk in this case is to "rev" the patient up more and make the sexual symptoms worse. Leave it to sexuality and dementia to bring out such oppositional treatment strategies. As of this writing, I know of no comparative studies. Sexuality in dementia is not a well-studied topic in general.

There is some data to suggest that some antihistamine/decongestants might reverse the sexual side effects of the SSRIs. While not likely of use for inappropriate sexual behaviors, this strategy might work for someone with dementia doing well on an SSRI yet struggling with inhibited sexual desire or functioning.

## WHAT ARE MOOD STABILIZERS?

In psychiatry, when one thinks of mood stabilizers, one generally considers the treatments for bipolar disorder. These include two general classes of medications. For the first, the U.S. Food and Drug Administration (FDA) indicates virtually all of the newer antipsychotics–the atypicals (see chapter 8, page 116)—for this purpose, as well as for the treatment of schizophrenia.

The other and more traditional class is the mood stabilizers. With the exception of lithium, which is seldom used in the elderly due to the kidney problems it can cause, these medications are used to control seizures. Given the chance for those with stroke disease to suffer seizures, and that unstable moods are often seen as being a core element of sexual behaviors in dementia patients, mood stabilizers are often a good medication to start with. Also, with the current trend toward trying to lower the use of antipsychotic medications in dementia patients, this is often the go-to medication group for other nonstroke dementia-related sexual problems as well.

By far, the most commonly used medication in this group is Depakote (divalproex sodium). This medication, in my experience, is generally well tolerated in lower doses; however, like any medication, side effects are more likely in the elderly than in younger patients—sedation and falls can occur. Also, there is a black box warning for liver failure, which is rarely seen. It is indicated for bipolar mania, not dementia-related mood issues. Thus using it for this purpose would be considered off label, which is a common practice that is generally considered safe in most instances.

Joe had dementia and trouble with loud verbal outbursts toward the nursing staff at a nursing home. His vulgarities, and requests for

***Mood Stabilizer Side Effects***

Nonantipsychotic mood stabilizers used for sexual behaviors in dementia and their most possible side effects are:

| Drug | Side Effect |
|---|---|
| Depakote (divalproex sodium) | tremor, liver failure |
| Lamictal (lamotrigine) | rash |
| Tegretol (carbamazepine) | anemia |
| Trileptal (oxycarbazepine) | low sodium |

sexual services, were going to get him discharged. An ex-army staff sergeant, he was a divorced alcoholic estranged from his children who reported that he'd been an "asshole" to them his entire life. I was asked to step in and get him under control. He was not on, and had not been on, any psychiatric medications as far as I could tell.

We started a course of Depakote 125 milligrams twice daily after checking his baseline liver function. Eventually he was getting a good result at 250 milligrams twice daily. Joe had zero side effects by week two and partial remission of his behaviors. The rest we figured was just Joe. As a rule, trying to fix personalities is not a goal of medication therapy.

## ANTIANXIETY MEDICATIONS

One of the most widely used substances in the world for anxiety is alcohol, and it happens that alcohol is often associated with sexual behaviors and situations. It is well known that, in many people, alcohol's effect allows for more social comfort and to some degree a release of inner impulses, such as sexuality. On the other hand, it is also known that sexual functioning and performance is diminished under the influence of alcohol.

While those with dementia are not, as a rule, a group with a high rate of current alcohol consumption, they are often given antianxiety medications to calm down. The effect of such medications (known as the benzodiazepines) on sexuality in dementia patients is similar to that of alcohol in others, that is, a relaxation of inhibitions and poorer sexual performance. From the standpoint of avoiding inappropriate sexual behaviors, the performance factor is not nearly as important as is the increased likelihood of allowing the behaviors to develop.

While it is true that these medications can be used successfully to stop any number of behaviors, including sexual ones, doing so occurs in doses high enough to cause sedation and lethargy. Short of end-of-life or palliative care, these are usually not considered to be acceptable side effects in the long run. As a rule, the benzodiazepines, or sedative hypnotics as they are also known, play a small role in the management of sexual behaviors in dementia patients other than a means to emergently stop a behavior that cannot otherwise be curtailed. Despite these concerns, benzodiazepines remain widely used across the United States as a solution for many kinds of distress in dementia patients. Such patients, while usually not ready or able to engage sexually themselves, may become vulnerable to predation by another patient or even a caregiver. The case of Cindy, which I learned about from a nurse friend, reminds me of that.

Cindy was a woman with moderate dementia who had been giving her assisted living facility a very difficult time with her behaviors. Her family and physician were in agreement that something to calm her was needed, and that something was Ativan three times a day. It worked. She was calmed but barely able to socialize and in her room much of the time. One day a staff nurse entered to find a man with a history of predation in the act of forcing her to give him oral sex. Cindy, slowed and confused, was unable to mount any sort of opposition. Just to be sure she was all right, she was sent to the ER to be checked. There it was discovered she had vaginal abrasions consistent with aggressive penetration. It was felt the same man was the perpetrator; however, he, ironically, was actually more confused than Cindy and unable to give further details. A treatment plan was developed, including getting Cindy off the Ativan, after which she became much more alert. In addition to environmental and behavioral approaches, a low dose of a mood stabilizer was started. It helped to manage her behavioral distress with less sedation.

***Commonly Used Antianxiety Drugs***

Benzodiazepines commonly used in dementia patients are:

- Ativan (lorazepam)
- Klonopin (clonazepam)
- Restoril (temazepam)
- Xanax (alprazolam)

## SEX, LIES, AND ANTIPSYCHOTICS

Let's call it a lot of misinformation. The antipsychotics are far from perfect. Side effects range from sedation to Parkinson's-like tremors to death. In fact, there is currently a black box warning for all of the atypical antipsychotics for an increased risk of death, as well as the development of heart irregularities and diabetes, in elderly dementia patients. But, despite good studies that refute this warning, it has led to a nationwide mandate to rid nursing homes of antipsychotics. More importantly, this class of medication is often useful to reverse the risks of death from agitation and psychosis, two severe risks not mentioned nearly as much as the warnings about the drugs. (As already stated in chapter 8, typical antipsychotics are older versions of the drugs versus the atypicals, or newer versions. The best-known typicals include Haldol (haloperidol) and Thorazine (chlorpromazine). Their packaging does not include black box warnings about increased risk of death in dementia patients. The typicals tend to cause more side effects than the newer atypicals, which is why the latter are used more often. The most well-known atypicals include Risperdal [risperidone], Seroquel [quetiapine], and Zyprexa [olanzapine]. Their packaging does include black box warnings.)

After the medical problems have been ruled out and the environmental and behavioral approaches have been exhausted, something must be done to treat the patients in distress or causing harm to themselves or others. Other drug options often fail. The troubles with Ativan are known, and while there are some other choices, such as Depakote or Prazosin—or even an antidepressant—what are the next choices if they don't work?

Put me on an island with 100 dementia patients and allow me three medications to help them survive until help arrives. One of the three would be an antipsychotic. The newer ones, the atypicals, are indicated for bipolar illness, schizophrenia, and even depression in two of the medications (Seroquel and Abilify). In low doses they often do alone what several other medications could not, which is treat psychosis, stabilize moods, and calm anxiety and agitation, all the while preserving critical activity level—*if* side effects are well managed.

In terms of sexual behaviors, this class of medications is not for all situations. Behaviors involving a psychosis (misinterpreting situations), or mania, or severely disorganized thinking are often calmed by a low dose antipsychotic, which inevitably works in part by blocking dopamine, the pleasure neurotransmitter.

Antipsychotics can lead to continuous physical and mental disruption like moving from ER to ER due to lack of stable placement, noncompliance with medical care, and falls from sedation due to Ativan. In extreme cases, the result can even be death. One should, in fact, never use an antipsychotic, or any medication for that matter, without balancing the risks. While the risk of death from the atypical antipsychotics has been reported to be low, it has appeared to be real and well documented in studies.

Other studies and even large recent presentations have refuted this risk. And I have seen such cases myself. In the end, there should be a balance, weighing all the risks with all the benefits.

Kim, for instance, had moderate dementia. He had come to a skilled nursing facility for rehabilitation care for an arm fracture after a fall. Used to living in a quiet setting with his spouse, he was clearly getting overly excited from all the busyness at the facility. He was elated, excited, delusional (thinking things that weren't real), and grabbing at a breast or bottom every chance he could. His wife was embarrassed. We discussed the medication options, including the risks and benefits, as all else seemed to be failing. Given his frank psychotic symptoms mixed in with the apparent mania, she agreed to a trial of Risperdal, an antipsychotic.

We started out at a super low dose (0.25milligrams twice daily) and went up from there. Kim stabilized nicely from his sexual behaviors at 0.5 milligrams twice daily, but we had a new problem. Kim, now with a tremor, was walking with a shuffling gait and leaning to one side. Mental status wise, he seemed blunted and flat. These were obvious extrapyramidal symptoms (EPS). This is the Parkinson's-like side effect that antipsychotic drugs can cause and is due to the dopamine blockade. (The "pyramids" are the corticospinal tract down the spinal cord that carries the major motor nerves. Some of the extra pyramidal nerves, outside the corticospinal tract, control fine motor movements. These nerves are disturbed in Parkinson's, or by the side effect of these drugs. All this is due to a lack of dopamine, which is blocked by the drug.)

The wife and I both agreed that this side effect was intolerable. When these side effects occur, and the decision is made to keep trying the antipsychotic approach, Seroquel is the next step. This is the medication given to psychotic Parkinson's patients. Rather, sedation and blood pressure issues are what need to be monitored. We stopped the Risperdal for 24 hours and started Seroquel at 12.5 milligrams, twice daily. The Parkinson's symptoms were gone after 48 hours. We gradually increased the Seroquel to 50 milligrams three times daily, which he tolerated well. (Schizophrenics and bipolar patients are often on 400 to 600 milligrams daily.)

Kim's inappropriate sexual behavior had vanished by week two, and he was calm and comfortable with an even mood. He was

### *Commonly Used Antipsychotics*

**Typical (older)**

- Haldol (haloperidol)
- Thorazine (chlorpromazine)

*(continued)*

***Commonly Used Antipsychotics (continued)***

**Atypical**

- Abilify (aripiprazole)
- Clozaril (clozapine)
- Geodon (ziprazidone)
- Invega (paliperidone)
- Risperdal (risperidone)
- Seroquel (quetiapine)
- Zyprexa (olanzapine)

sleeping and eating well and participated in all activities with little or no daytime sedation. Over the next year we were able to wean him off the Seroquel with no recurrence of the behaviors.

## HORMONAL THERAPY

The effects of hormone therapy on dementia have been the subject of research. Interestingly, decreased testosterone levels are generally found in male Alzheimer's sufferers compared with control patients. A review of the literature supports this finding, as do other studies. While one review suggests that there is not enough evidence to promote testosterone replacement in men for the same purpose, there is evidence that testosterone does reduce the secretion of the toxic B amyloid proteins found in Alzheimer's dementia. A study of testosterone replacement in Alzheimer's patients showed a significant improvement in quality of life, including energy, well-being, and relationships, but no effect on the cognitive decline. In spite of this, reviews of castrated men do not suggest an increase in dementia might be predicted by a "low T" hypothesis.

Even women have been the subjects of testosterone replacement to prevent cognitive decline. However, the results do not support the use of testosterone replacement for such a purpose. The fact that there are more women with dementia is felt to have more to do with them living longer than on lower testosterone levels.

Still, the idea of estrogen replacement in women to prevent cognitive decline has drawn considerable interest. While mention is made in one study that estrogen replacement in women is controversial and uncertain for the purpose of dementia prevention, there are studies that clearly show such estrogen replacement therapy to be beneficial in reducing the frequency of dementia. These studies are somewhat dated, but a more recent article provides an interesting review that is very supportive of the neuroprotective estrogen therapy for Alzheimer's disease. There are articles that suggest that this neuroprotection likely involves several different factors including antioxidation effects on neurons and the prevention of atherosclerosis, the fatty plaques that build inside arteries.

Yet controversy remains regarding the use of estrogen replacement, in part due to the medical risks, such as cancer. Also, reviews suggest that estrogen therapy may in fact not prevent Alzheimer's disease in women at all.

Nonetheless, since testosterone is the hormonal force behind human sex drive for both men and women, it makes sense to try and diminish it as a means of stabilizing sexual behaviors. Medroxyprogesterone acetate (Provera), a synthetic form of progesterone, Cyproterone (the drug names Androcur and Cyprostat) and estrogen has been used for this purpose as each has the ability to diminish testosterone production.

Provera can be given either orally or in an injection every three months, and is, in my experience, the most common hormonal treatment used for sexual behaviors in dementia patients. Its use as a means of chemical castration in sexual offenders underscores the potential ethical concerns and sensitivities surrounding its use in dementia patients.

Most commonly, this treatment strategy in dementia patients comes as a long-term solution for continuing problems involving predatory behavior that has not been successfully treated by any other means. I am reminded of Bill, a 72-year-old, who was a resident of a facility I consulted at that specialized in the worst of the behavior cases. To say the least, it was an interesting mix of dementia with chronic mental illness.

Bill had a lengthy history of sexual behaviors with both staff and patients. My understanding is that he had always been a strange man with issues when it came to his interactions with people and suggestive of a personality disorder. As his stroke disease progressed, the point came when he was diagnosed with dementia. He bounced from facility to facility, eventually becoming recognized as a "dirty old man." He did have a daughter, but she wanted nothing to do with him. Due to that, he had an appointed guardian.

Bill's sexual behaviors—grabbing, making comments, and fondling patients—eventually presented themselves in full color about a month or two after admission to the facility. I discussed the options with the guardian, who told me, "He's been on everything since I've been working with him. Nothing has worked. He's kind of a pervert, you know?" After examining Bill, it was determined that there was no psychosis or unstable mood present. None of the behavioral approaches worked. He seemed to be a candidate for hormonal therapy.

We started oral Provera, eventually switching over to the injection. After several weeks, Bill showed a marked reduction in his sexually oriented behavior with no apparent side effects to the medication. He was able to stay at the facility and became an asset as a member of the community.

### *Medication Approaches to Sexual Behaviors*

**Passive**

1. Review all medications looking for recent changes that coincide with behaviors
2. Stop or reduce a suspected culprit medication
3. Monitor and assess the need for an alternative
4. Long-term use of an antidementia medication may delay onset of behaviors. They include:
   a. Aricept (donepezil)
   b. Exelon (rivastigmine)
   c. Namenda (memantine)
   d. Razadyne (galantamine)

**Active**

1. Start a medication targeting the cause of sexual behaviors:
   a. Depakote (divalproex)
   b. An antipsychotic
2. Start a medication directly targeting sexual behaviors:
   a. SSRI (may cause mania)
   b. Hormonal therapy
3. Start a medication targeted at sedation (extreme measures/comfort care):
   a. Ativan (lorazepam)
   b. Morphine sulfate

## AN INEXACT SCIENCE

There are so many variables that one can never be sure what will, or will not, work on unexpected sexual behaviors. There are other medications that have been tried, at times successfully, that are as disparate in function as those I have mentioned. Propranolol, a beta-blocker, is a blood pressure medication that blocks the beta receptors of epinephrine while Prazosin, also a blood pressure medication, is an alpha receptors blocker. Cimetidine blocks histamine receptors. An even wider variety of environmental and behavioral approaches have been put forth, some successful, some not.

The many complex variables range from known biochemical sexual mechanisms, such as the frontal lobe, the limbic system, testosterone, or dopamine, to the talents of the staff and to the personalities of the patients. All the while, treating the sexual behaviors is paramount to everyone involved, including families, caregivers, the victims, administrators, state regulators, and most importantly, each patient. After all is said and done, hopefully a balance will have been struck between treating an illness, protecting those in harm's way, and allowing the patient to continue on with the fullest access to his or her humanness.

CHAPTER TEN

# Where We Go from Here

The number of dementia cases is increasing. The older the population gets, the more dementia will be diagnosed. Our brains simply have physical limits. And while it is expected that people will lose mental, as well as physical abilities as they age, the reality is that dementia begins while people may still be healthy. In that case, the numbers of people with the disease are much greater than believed. A recent newspaper article related studies discussed at an Alzheimer's conference in Boston. The studies "showed that people with some types of cognitive concerns were more likely to have Alzheimer's pathology in their brains, and to develop dementia later." In a potentially far-reaching development, researchers identified what they are calling "subjective cognitive decline." What this means is that what people report about themselves regarding what they perceive as poorer memory and diminished cognitive skills should be taken seriously, even if they don't show symptoms of dementia. The people who reported their worry about their mental decline were, sadly, right. Their brains were found to contain amyloids, the Alzheimer's-related proteins.

What these findings will lead to, what kind of tests or, hopefully, treatments will result, is presently unknown. Perhaps it will lead to a shift in how we view aging, and, in particular, the connection between aging and sexuality.

## THE GREAT AMERICAN CONTRADICTION

It's a picture that Americans embrace: solid marriage, good job, three kids, a dog, and maybe even a white picket fence around the house. Then, after decades pass, you watch the grandkids as you grow old together. It is assumed that the two of you are happy, even if you are both somewhat forgetful. You slow down as the years go by, but the relationship stays strong. As you walk together, holding hands, you are the symbol of enduring love.

But there is one part of this scenario that is denied. Though it is never discussed, or even thought about much by others, sexual attraction remains. You both still get a little frisky under the pile of comforters you sleep under each night. You are hardly alone, yet this important and ongoing part of aging is virtually denied in our society, just because you are old. Without acknowledging that sex continues throughout life, how will it be possible to really understand that sexuality lives on in those with dementia?

In America, we seem to want to see the aging process less and less. It is an airbrush culture where our lives are seen through a sugarcoated lens. The message, and a not very subtle one, is that one is supposed to live long but look young and sexy.

Sexual attraction and activity is focused on the young and the young looking. And though being 60 years old and up isn't the same as it was in our grandparents' time (how many grandmothers went to a gym on a regular basis, and how many grandfathers knew their triglyceride counts?), there is a widespread assumption that as we age we lose our sexual allure and desire. The combination of getting old and being sexually active is pretty much dismissed, if not joked about or regarded as something downright icky.

In contrast, the industries that promote youth hammer the message that looking young, or at least younger, is vital to being a sexual being. To that end, companies target age-conscious boomers. Related spending by the boomers is expected to reach $115 billion annually by 2015. This figure includes everything from antiaging creams to cosmetic surgeries.

After all, who doesn't want to look and feel as good as they can at any age? Still, while there is much to be said about taking care of yourself, it is naïve, if not self-defeating, to believe that looks and sexuality cannot be separated.

Bombarded by advertising and media, we buy into an image of youth equated with sex and yet privately smile at aging couples who show their engagement with one another. It is a mystery to me why our culture doesn't focus more on the positive and make this particular and special aspect of aging something to realistically look forward to. The obvious advantage of being older and romantic is maturity and experience, which, taken together, create more meaningful relationships.

What I find intriguing is that, with the exception of erectile dysfunction (ED)–related medications, there is little information or help about sexuality as we age. It's time we saw this campaign for what it is. The secondary pitch is that these medications are not for sexual issues in aging couples. The foremost message is that taking these drugs will keep you young looking and vital. That's what the fit and attractive actors and models are selling. They don't look like aging people with medical concerns.

ED, however, is a serious medical symptom that is directly related to a sex and aging issue, namely atherosclerotic disease, the fatty plaques on the inside of our arteries. Atherosclerosis, because it affects blood flow through the body, results in strokes and dementia, congestive heart failure and heart attacks, peripheral vascular disease in the legs, and chronic renal insufficiency in the kidneys. My estimate is that one-third of the deaths in the United States are related to atherosclerosis, based upon the Centers for Disease Control statistics (there are no actual numbers on atherosclerosis per se).

Yet what gets advertised the most, despite all the press on health concerns, is the effect of atherosclerotic disease on the penis, although the underlying cause is never mentioned. Some advertisements mention that ED is related to hypertension or diabetes, but they don't explain why. Nonetheless, there is general legal speak, as in, "Ask your doctor if it's okay for you to have sex." Then the ads go back to the promise of sex between the attractive, fit actors.

ED represents a condition that kills many men. Yet we don't see real aging people with medical dilemmas enjoying their sexuality. Instead, the advertising reinforces the message that good-looking people who look very healthy can still have sex.

Apparently the women in the ads, who appear to be about as old as, or slightly younger than, the men, don't have any problems or complaints. That in itself is odd, since postmenopausal women experience atrophic vaginitis, which can be treated with either topical or systemic estrogen and/or lubricants. Although it may be less related to atherosclerotic changes, it is no less important of a condition relative to sexual activity.

Overall, what is missing is the embracing of the realities of aging. People get old. When they do, their bodies change, inside and out. Looking different, understanding that injuries will take longer to heal than they did when a person was younger, thinking about life in a new, challenging way: all these considerations, and many more, seem to be secondary to how one looks. But perhaps the biggest insult to our aging population is the refusal to accept that many older people want to maintain their sex lives as long as they can.

## SEXUALITY IS A HEALTHY PART OF GROWING OLDER

I have polled, spoken to, and interviewed many groups and individuals, and the answer is always the same: Sexuality does persist into the later years. It takes different forms and magnitudes, but it does continue. Not only do I see this happening, I hear about it from other medical and social professionals who work with the elderly.

Research also bears this out. The website of the American Psychological Association includes studies regarding aging and sex, including cultural issues, all of which support sex and aging. In its "Aging and Human Sexuality Resource Guide," the Association makes its position clear. In the Introduction, Dr. Antonette M. Zeiss writes, "We don't discuss sexuality enough when considering the lives of older adults ... However, it is not easy for health professionals in training to find information to learn more about aging and sexuality, once they have realized how important this topic is. This website helps to solve that problem." To that end, the website lists many articles that address sexual activity and its related concerns and function among older men and women.

It is known that a general lessening of libido with age occurs and is biologically determined. There is a drop in levels of hormones, and thus a decline of sexual urge. But a decline doesn't mean less than zero. Much of the evidence points to continued sexuality in later years, despite lesser intensity due to biological changes. Also, studies suggest that the ratio between affection and physical sex leans more toward affection in the elderly.

The primary reason for this may well be that in later life we no longer need to reproduce. But to suggest that the only reason we have sex, the most extreme form of pleasure and intimacy, is solely for reproduction seems simplistic. In fact, since we generally become more self-aware as we age, the continuation of pleasure and intimacy makes sense. Regular sex is also associated with less depression and anxiety and more medical stability. On the social side, it is well documented, particularly for men, that being in a sexual relationship leads to better health and longevity, as well as a lower suicide rate. For women, the benefits are greater on the emotional, rather than the physical, side. These differences are minor, however, compared with the wealth of physical and emotional benefits of sex for both partners.

There are many reasons for wanting closeness with another person. Whether it is a craving for intimacy, a fear of being alone, a celebration of life, or a victory over cheating death, older people experience a range of sexual feelings, just as they did all their lives.

Why would anyone want to give that up, if they don't have to do so, just because they are older?

## AN AGING POPULATION WITH A CHANGING ATTITUDE

More than three million American boomers turn 55 every year, and currently the population of those over 65 tops 35 million. That is a significant contrast with the population of less than 100 years ago, when the average age of death for a man was 40. In 1930, there were only seven million people categorized as old, making up just over 5 percent of the population. Now 10,000 people sign up for Medicare every day, and the long-term care industry has a lot of willing participants.

The boomers have a propensity for stretching themselves physically, to get as much out of their bodies as they can for as long as possible. This is likely a side effect of the longevity and improved health care we now enjoy. Nonetheless, the boomers are next in line to feel the heat of aging. Those bodies they like to stretch will, at some point, fail to live up their standards. The boomers are in a state of flux, transitioning from the lie that American advertising has sold them and the reality of getting old.

But the boomers also read and seek information. They discuss their own issues and may even wonder about the possibility of romance and sex with a partner changed by dementia. After all, many are watching their parents go through those life-altering challenges right now.

It makes sense that a continuing sex life will be a goal for many, dementia or not. Add in the desire to connect emotionally and discuss their dilemma openly, and you have a huge population with no desire to bow to societal pressure to act in an expected way.

In the process of transitioning into the reality of aging, my expectation—and hope—would be for the boomers to lead the way toward a new awareness, not just for themselves but for others who follow after them. We all need something to lean on as we face mortality. For many, religion is vital in that role. But whether one is religious or not, someone to share the pains and fears with seems vital as well. The point is that real connections are not formed with electronic devices; they are formed with another living being who can return feelings.

That's exactly what I saw with Barney.

## A NEW AWARENESS

Barney had troubles. He was in his 50s and was tired of his job. He was also tired of his wife, Sheila. He still felt he loved her, but it was more of a companionship. Having no children, the couple generally spent each evening in separate parts of their large home. She watched "chick flicks" as he put it. He, unbeknownst to her, secretly surfed the Internet for pornography night after night. This had literally gone on for several years, until one night he heard a thud coming from the kitchen on the floor below. Barney ran downstairs to find his wife sprawled out on the floor, in the midst of a seizure.

The next day, in the ICU, Sheila remained unconscious. An MRI scan revealed that a large ballooning aneurysm had ruptured from a major artery in the brain. This was the equivalent of a massive stroke that involved a large area of the brain.

I met the couple a year later, each in a separate struggle. Sheila was confused and frustrated. She was partially paralyzed and unable to get words out. Barney, in stark contrast, was nothing short of engaged. He was there, day after day after work. He knew her medications and was aware of her needs. He developed a constructive relationship with the staff and did what he could to assist them with her care.

I took him aside after I was asked to see her for her anxiety. He told me the story, including what had transpired with him over the past year. "We were on two separate tracks," he began. "God forbid this should happen to anyone, but I love her more than I ever thought I could love anyone, and she knows it. They even let us spend a little private time together—you know what I mean. It's not a guilt trip. What happened wasn't my fault. It's just one of those things that changed us. I realized what I was missing in our relationship. It's awful that Sheila has to cope with her condition for the rest of her life—but I am coping with it, too. I never knew I would feel the way I do. But I'm so glad that I do."

## ANOTHER APPROACH TO SEX AND DEMENTIA

I am still struck over the current struggle we Americans maintain, relative to other cultures, with the concept of sex and dementia.

A recent story I came across on YouTube, and elsewhere on the Internet, concerned the impact of Australian sex workers on dementia care. The discussion, generated on *Insight*, a progressive Australian television program, demonstrated a comfort with the subject of sexuality and dementia in that country. For one, the idea and partial acceptance of the "sex worker" concept as a means of servicing the needs of, and providing comfort to, those with dementia is something that would be met with quite a bit more controversy in the United States. The mere existence of that conversation is lacking in America. Secondly, it is clear from the conversation that in Australia there is more openness in general when discussing the emotional and physical needs, including sexual ones, of those with dementia. In effect, the afflicted are treated like anyone else.

In one particular case, a woman discussed openly, in front of an audience, her recognition of the sexual needs of her 93-year-old father who had dementia. She hired a sex worker to meet those needs. The result appeared to benefit his mood and sense of well-being. It would be quite an advancement to see such societal acceptance of the sexual needs of dementia patients in the United States.

Things are changing, but it's a slow process. Searching the current literature reveals that the majority of the focus on dementia care is in making the diagnosis and managing the behaviors. While dementia is being diagnosed more often in the primary care office, the focus still seems to be on the bits and pieces, such as starting Aricept, giving education about not driving, or not leaving the stove when something is cooking. Unfortunately, the emotional issues holding the patient together—the relationship dynamics, sexual needs, and living situational planning for the future—are not being addressed.

## WHAT CAN BE DONE

There will always be the need for long-term care. Dementia is a progressive disease that will culminate in high-care needs and behavioral challenges, including those that are sexual in nature. Hopefully, changes will occur in long-term care where more interest will take place when it comes to the day-to-day lives of those with dementia. Staff and facilities will be better trained to recognize sexual behavioral challenges and the sexual needs that their clients are expressing and find ways to meet them. My guess is that, ultimately, more facilities will become experienced with dealing with developing relationships between clients.

At present, many of the larger companies dealing with long-term care have their own development staffs. They consist of knowledgeable nurses and social workers dedicated to training others on the sexual needs and complexities found in dementia patients. Smaller facilities or companies rely upon independent experts (like me) or other staff in departments such as ours who deal with dementia-related behaviors regularly.

The current federal regulations address a need for dementia patients in long-term care and generally mandate access to the fullest life that is both possible and practical. My hope would be that the future would bring more specifics when it comes to sexuality. The existing vagueness appears to avoid the complex issue of sexuality and dementia and leaves facilities and families to sort out a lot on their own.

I believe that detailing levels of sexual behavior in those with dementia, with the regulations outlining what is or is not acceptable, makes sense. Doing so would help to develop policies, procedures, training, and awareness that would lead everyone affected by dementia, including medical personnel and caregivers, closer to accomplishing the original goal of the regulations. That goal is access to the fullest life experience possible for all involved. Specific concerns should include privacy, verbal language, physical acts, and relationships.

For families and partners, my desire is that you and your loved ones will be protected by a health care system that will understand what all of you are struggling with. It will be a system that knows how to address sexual and relationship concerns and is continuously available for consultation, for instance a case management model rather than a follow-up appointment in six months.

For professionals, my wish would be that dementia becomes a sought-after field to specialize in. This should be reflected in research studies and grants as well. I believe that pharmaceutical companies looking at curing a disease fund too much research in that particular area. More studies and grants that delve into the relationship dynamics of dementia, as well as into the issues of abuse and neglect and how to counter them, are needed.

But significant changes will only come after a shift in the way society views sex and dementia.

## DEMENTIA AND TECHNOLOGY: NOT SUCH ODD BEDFELLOWS

We are in the midst of a technological revolution. Looking at the bigger timescale, one could argue it has been ongoing since the beginning of the 20th century. Clean water, improved sanitation, antibiotics, and much more, have resulted in longevity. And with longevity has come dementia.

A case might be made that dementia is an unintentional consequence—a side effect—of technology. Is this bad? Perhaps we really weren't supposed to live this long. Maybe dying from childbirth or plague or appendicitis might be more in line with the true human condition as it had been for the past thousands of years.

Yet more and more, technology is being used to prompt the memories of those with dementia. This is being used to optimize caregiving as well as moods and anxiety levels. Some work is being done exploring the use of computers in assisting those with dementia in their relationships with caregivers. Think about it: who hasn't been caught up emotionally by a smell or a song or a visual cue like a photograph? By designing a computerized profile specific to the history of someone based upon their age, ethnicity, and cultural background, a host of cues might be generated to serve a confused patient in a variety of ways. It could calm, act as a reminder or cue, or entertain in a way specific to that person.

It might not be too much of a stretch to imagine how the use of this technology might spark memories and contribute to the quality in an ongoing romantic relationship. Another use might be something a spouse could introduce to calm an escalating situation. This might be in the form of technology-based games, tasks, or images.

## A NEW MORALITY

As we move forward into this strange new world of advancing technology and increased awareness of diseases like Alzheimer's, the question has been raised about what this might mean from an ethical point of view relative to traditional views of marriage and the vows against infidelity therein. John Portmann, a professor of religious studies at the University of Virginia, writes about the morality of relationships and dementia. His view is that we are on the brink of a major shift in the norm when it comes to monogamy in marriage or relationships by virtue of the vast numbers in the aging population who may soon be facing life with a partner with dementia. He believes that a general liberalization of social views across our country may well lead to acceptance of relationships outside the bonds of marriage.

In contrast to the cases where two unrelated people in a facility who have sex with each other cause chaos and result in separation, more and more I hear of cases where there is no chaos, and sexual relations are being allowed without incident.

The question here is whether or not, from a societal point of view, there is an ethical change on the horizon. Will the concept of "Until death do us part" get a new meaning? Tim and Allison remind me of this dilemma.

Tim and Alison had been married 30 years up to the point where she developed Alzheimer's disease at age 52. I knew them personally and still remember the day Tim told me Alison had been seen by a neurologist and diagnosed with dementia. I asked him to bring her to me for an examination, and, sure enough, she had all the signs and symptoms, including the memory loss and a superficial pleasantness as though trying her best to gloss it all over.

It was heartbreaking for me, and I would think disastrous for them, but he just seemed to take it all in stride. They were very religious. Tim indicated that Alison's illness was all a part of God's plan, and that it would all be okay. I felt he was in denial. I worried that he wasn't going to plan, and that the magnitude of the situation was going to hit him like a ton of bricks down the road. Fortunately, Tim and I saw each other often enough that I could keep tabs on him. I would ask, "Did you see the financial planner? Have you got some part-time help coming in at home? Has Alison been enrolled in the research program at the University or started the day program yet?" No matter how many questions I asked, Tim seemed to be on top of the issues over the next five years as Alison slowly slipped away.

And then one day Tim dropped a bombshell. He was seeing someone else. The one area that I didn't ask a whole lot about, that I wished I had, was how things were between the two of them. It wasn't as if doing so would have made a difference necessarily, but the disclosure was shocking because Alison and Tim were long-time friends of mine. Then I realized that Tim had his own difficult journey to take, and where that led him was something that was very private.

The new lady was someone he had met a couple of years before. They had been dating for a year, and it was now serious, so much so that they were planning to marry. I was entering new territory in terms of how I felt. Still, I had to admit that it was understandable for him to form another serious relationship. Tim's sexual and romantic needs had been unmet for some time by Alison, who was already in the advanced stages of her illness.

Tim went into more detail about his plan. It was well thought out with the help of a noted Seattle elder law attorney. By divorcing his wife he would be able to essentially make her appear poor enough to be placed on Medicaid, which would allow her access to considerable long-term care expenses. He would acquire 100 percent of the assets in the settlement—they were not rich by any standard—but with the agreement he would then put 50 percent of the assets into a trust that their two children would manage and use to supplement the Medicaid. Nothing about it was impulsive, not even his relationship or plan to marry. He had planned to the *n*th degree.

## THE BLURRY LINE IN THE SAND

In the future, we don't know where societal, religious, and ethical views will stand relative to moving on from relationships with dementia patients. This already is not a rare event, and across the country one can legally obtain a no-fault divorce from someone with dementia as long as the patient is represented to protect his or her interests. However, the reverse is not so simple. While a guardian protects those interests, someone who has been deemed incompetent has no possibility of obtaining a divorce should he or she desire it. And what about a dementia patient who does not yet have a guardian, or someone who has not been deemed incompetent by a judge? The word *incompetent* is a legal term. (In my practice, I have given an opinion about a person's capacity. That opinion, in turn, can be used in a competency hearing.)

It is often a different matter in a situation where someone has enacted their power of attorney by virtue of a letter a physician might have written expressing an opinion as to the patient's *incapacity* to make decisions. This happens in the majority of cases and is a much blurrier line in the sand. This situation, like that of the healthier partner's leaving, could raise eyebrows as well. It certainly did in a case I well remember—that of Hank. What a fireball he had always been.

Hank was admitted to our inpatient service for a psychosis and unstable mood related to his dementia. His son and daughter, a physician and a nurse, had done all they could to protect their medically ill mother from their father, who, amidst his confusion, had been causing her a great deal of distress with demands for everything from sex to money. The children were joint medical powers of attorney for him and felt they only needed a letter from me stating that their father was unable to make his own decisions. I wrote the letter, which I felt was consistent with the psychiatric examination. At the same time, I held out hope that he might be able to regain his independence with treatment, as it was more the mania and psychosis (each, I felt, borne out of the dementia) rather than his confusion that was causing most of the trouble.

Hank partially complied with treatment and calmed somewhat over the next two weeks. It was agreed by all, except Hank, that he would be discharged to a memory care assisted living facility. When confronted with this decision he eventually complied.

At the memory care facility, Hank wasted no time in taking matters into his own hands. He stopped all his medications and demanded a second opinion and then a third. All agreed with me that he lacked enough understanding of his situation to make his own decisions. The facility was anxious to rehospitalize him because they were concerned that he was making enough sense to be released and didn't want to be responsible for holding him against his will. Hank found the solution to his problem, namely a lawyer.

It wasn't long until the lawyer and his new client took steps to delegitimize the power of attorney and threaten the facility. Holding a person against his will without a legal structure, such as a power of attorney or guardianship, is not allowed. A facility cannot detain a person without calling for the state or county to detain him involuntarily. Because Hank was not deemed to be a threat to himself or others, he was declined for involuntary detainment, and he was released on his own recognizance. The daughter had become so sickened by the affair that she lost 20 pounds and was hospitalized for depression. The son began drinking again after 10 years of sobriety. Neither of them had either the health or the interest to fight their father.

Hank's first steps were to buy a car, find a new home, and file for divorce. He ended up getting 50 percent of the assets while expressing no interest in his wife's health or emotional concerns. This, of course, only sickened the children further. He filed a complaint about me with the state department of health for orchestrating an offensive against him; it took months to untangle. To this day, Hank is living alone, estranged from his family and driving a car.

In the future there will be more and more people with some degree of confusion who will be trying to exercise their rights and likely finding lawyers to help them. Who knows? These kinds of situations might even become a legal specialty.

## INTO THE UNEXPECTED FUTURE

What can you to do as you enter the unexpected future? How can you be realistic, minimize the risk, and move forward with a rewarding relationship? I asked this of a couple I know, Lenny and Rene. Both are healthy. They've been married 22 years and have two teen girls. They eat a healthy diet and get plenty of exercise. They are as in love and romantic together as ever. They both came from families with longevity. They are not religious, but would each admit they would call out for God if dying. They have a joint motto for dealing with problems—analyze, minimize, and move on. I interviewed them separately and asked them how dementia might impact their marriage.

Rene: *Dementia. I think it would be me. I hope it would be me. I just feel that way. I love Lenny so much and want to protect him, even if it means me getting sick. I'm not sure what that would be like. Would I just go away mentally? Could we still have a relationship? It's the memory, right? It goes away. Then how would I even know it was him? Oh my God. I could be with other men and think it was him? He'd still love me, but he would find someone, eventually. I don't blame him for that, but he'd need that after a while. Would I be a mess? And need cleaning? The girls could help with that. He'd fall apart. I want it to be me.*

Lenny: *I don't even want to think about it. Don't even want to go there. Don't we all get a little trouble with our memory when we get to 90, like our grandparents? They all got along and stayed together. We'll probably be like them. Our parents are going to be like that.*

Many people feel that they are right or that they know what they will do. To that I say, be careful. I say that even to those with strong religious views, couples with marriages that have lasted for decades, and to those with vast medical knowledge. Time and time again, my experience has shown me that events have a way of changing things in ways no one could have predicted. This is all the more of a surprise in situations involving love and romance because of the promise, the certainty, and the importance of these aspects of our lives. The divorce rates already demonstrate how unpredictable relationships are, even before dementia enters the picture. Add an illness to a relationship where a partner has pulled away and changed in such a way that he or she might no longer seem to be the same person, and nothing is certain.

Betty and Maurice certainly underscore that. Betty was recently admitted to our inpatient service for agitation when I heard their story from their only child, Eve. They had always had a stormy marriage filled with fights and threats of separation. They divorced and went their separate ways when Eve was twelve. In the coming years they each remarried relatively successfully, giving Eve a set of stepparents that she became fond of. In later years, though, these stepparents died, just as Maurice and Betty were each slipping into the throes of dementia.

Eve kept them separated in two different memory care facilities, but eventually she brought Betty over to see Maurice for a visit. To Eve's surprise, they reconnected in a loving and somewhat passionate way that could never have been predicted. To this day they live separately, which was partially the source of Betty's agitation, but cannot seem to wait for the next visit together when, with no fighting, they spend their time together like the loving and lasting couple they never were.

I asked Eve, "Do you think they recognize one another?" She replied, "It's foggy some days, but they respect and admire each other like they never could before. In some odd way, I feel like we now have the family we never did. I'd never wish dementia on anyone, but maybe there's a lesson here for all of us."

### *Six Steps to Plan for Sexuality and Dementia*

The unpleasant reality is that dementia in general is probably underdiagnosed because it is relatively low on the medical radar. In addition, there is the family/spouse denial factor.

*(continued)*

***Six Steps to Plan for Sexuality and Dementia (continued)***

I believe that young as well as middle-aged couples should factor the possibility of dealing with dementia into their long-range plans. You can:

1. Be real with the odds of getting dementia. Be aware of the following:
   a. Family history—genetics
   b. Environment—alcohol, exercise, nutrition, smoking
   c. Health risks—diabetes, high cholesterol, and hypertension.
2. Know what it means to get dementia and the caregiving impact.
3. Get legal documents in order, including a will and advanced directives, such as the possibility of authorizing a partner or spouse to protect themselves and any children, as well as you, from yourself.
4. Talk about it from time to time with your partner.
5. Talk about it from time to time with yourself.
6. Form a long-term care plan, including long-term care insurance, if possible.

## CONNECTIONS ALWAYS MATTER

I've treated thousands of people with dementia. Rarely is someone truly alone in her or his disease, without a family or friend or someone who cares. And even those who are alone yearn, in their own ways, to be connected and to be touched.

For the professional caregiver, there is a degree of control. These people bring experience, training, and professional development, which, when brought forth, forms a powerful tool to connect emotionally and yet also therapeutically. For the lover, however, there is only the experience, which is too long a time and too painful for words. For those with the disease, rational thinking mixes with love like oil and water. The best that can be hoped for is a lasting suspension—some oil here and some water there. With that, no one can know for sure how he or she will react initially to a love partner with dementia.

Down the road, thoughtful choices borne out of that very love may be contradictory and controversial.

But connections can stay open if we look for them. Initially, unique openings may present themselves through the breakage of social inhibitions. With time, apathy and confusion will dim the light that once was. Still, those stricken so severely will be there, waiting more and more deeply inside, to be reached by someone who cares.

# Notes

## CHAPTER THREE

p. 28: *Research has reported the effects...* Elmer Goudsmit et al., "The Supraoptic and Paraventricular Nuclei of the Human Hypothalamus in Relation to Sex, Age and Alzheimer's Disease," *Neurobiology of Aging 11*, no. 5 (1990): 529–36.

p. 31: *In my own research, I've noticed a 30 to 50 percent prevalence rate...*Douglas Wornell, "The Prevalence of Pseudobulbar Affect in 6 Neurological Conditions," *Prism Registry*, Avanir Pharmaceuticals PRNewswire, (September 20, 2012)

p. 38: *It may also occur in some variants...* Shawn J. Kile et al., "Alzheimer Abnormalities of the Amygdala with Klüver–Bucy Syndrome Symptoms An Amygdaloid Variant of Alzheimer's Disease," *Archives of Neurology 66*, no. 1 (2009): 125–29.

p. 39: *There is a trend toward studies...the disease, in some studies...* Christine L. Carter et al., "Sex and Gender Differences in Alzheimer's Disease: Recommendations for Future Research," *Journal of Women's Health 21*, no. 10 (2012): 1018–23.

p. 39: *Other studies found no difference...* Brenda L. Plassman et al., "Prevalence of Dementia in the United States: The Aging, Demographics, and Memory Study," *Neuroepidemiology 29*, no. 1–2 (2007): 125–32; Annemieke Ruitenberg, "Incidence of Dementia: Does Gender Make a Difference?" *Neurobiology of Aging 22*, no. 4 (2001): 575–80.

p. 39: *Another study that reported hypersexual behavior…* Hugh Series and Pilar Dégano, "Hypersexuality in Dementia," *Advances in Psychiatric Treatment 11*, no. 6 (2005): 424–431.

p. 39: *For example, "social impropriety" was found to be…* B. R. Ott, K. L. Lapane, and G. Gambassi, "Gender Differences in the Treatment of Behavior Problems in Alzheimer's Disease. SAGE Study Group. Systemic Assessment of Geriatric Drug Use Via Epidemiology," *Neurology, 54,* no. 2 (2000): 427–32.

p. 39: *and another reported a drastically higher incidence…* Kannayiram Alagiakrishnan et al., "Sexually Inappropriate Behaviour in Demented Elderly People," *Postgraduate Medical Journal 81,* no. 957 (2005): 463–66. doi:10.1136/pgmj.2004.028043

## CHAPTER SIX

p. 76: *It has been reported that…* Brenda L. Plassman et al., "Prevalence of Dementia in the United States: The Aging, Demographics, and Memory Study," *Neuroepidemiology 29,* no. 1–2 (2007): 125–32.

p. 78: *It is known from studies, for example…* K. Jellinger et al., "Clinicopathological Analysis of Dementia Disorders in the Elderly," *Journal of Neurological Sciences* 95, no. 3 (1990): 239–58; Columbia University Medical Center, "Link Between Alzheimer's and Stroke Illuminated," *ScienceDaily* (March 19, 2008).

p. 81: *A recently completed study demonstrated…* Laura F. DeFina et al., "The Association between Midlife Cardiorespiratory Fitness Levels and Later-Life Dementia: A Cohort Study." *Annals of Internal Medicine 158,* no. 3 (2013): 162–68.

p. 82: *Another study reported that a slowing…* J. Eric Ahlskog et al., "Physical Exercise as a Preventive or Disease-Modifying Treatment of Dementia and Brain Aging," Mayo Clinic Proceedings *86,* no. 9 (2011): 876–84.

## CHAPTER SEVEN

p. 99: *A recent report by…a UCLA assistant professor of neurology…* John Darrell Van Horn et al., "Mapping Connectivity Damage in the Case of Phineas Gage," *PLoS ONE* 7, no. 5 (2012): doi:10.1371/journal.pone.0037454

p. 102: *It is well known that personality changes…* Alfredo Ardila, "Head Trauma: Neurobehavioral Aspects," Clinical Summary, *MedLink*

*Neurology*, original publication 1994, updated 2012. www.medlink.com/medlinkcontent.asp?page=cip&uid=MLT00087

p. 105: *A review of the literature...* D. Mittal et al., "Worsening of Post-Traumatic Stress Disorder Symptoms with Cognitive Decline: Case Series," *Journal of Geriatric Psychiatry and Neurology 14*, no. 1 (2001): 17–20.

p. 105: *An Australian newsletter discusses this relatively...* Haley Clark and Kirsty Duncanson, "An Interview with Adelle Williams, Communication Change Observation Respect and Dignity Aged Care Training Specialist," Australian Institute for Family Studies Newsletter, *Aware 24* (2010): 9–12.

## CHAPTER EIGHT

p. 114: *Despite the obvious inclination to use testosterone...* Stephen E. Borst and Thomas Mulligan, "Testosterone Replacement Therapy for Older Men," *Journal of Clinical Interventions in Aging 2*, no. 4 (2007): 561–66.

p. 114: *Estrogen replacement therapy (ERT) has found a place...* P. M. Sarrel, "Effects of Hormone Replacement Therapy on Sexual Psychophysiology and Behavior in Postmenopause," *Journal of Women's Health and Gender-Based Medicine 9*, Supp. 1 (2000): S25–S32.

p. 114: *However, other studies demonstrate that testosterone...* P. Sarrel, B. Dobay, and B. Witta, "Estrogen and Estrogen–Androgen Replacement in Postmeopausal Women Dissatisfied with Estrogen-Only Therapy. Sexual Behavior and Neuroendocrine Responses." *Journal of Reproductive Medicine 43*, no. 10 (1998): 847–56.

p. 114: *Studies report that elderly men...* R. D. Abbott et al., "Serum Estradiol and Risk of Stroke in Elderly Men," *Neurology 68*, no. 8 (2007): 563–68.

p. 114: *There is also a clear suppression...* M. Kwan, J. VanMaasdam, and J. M. Davidson, "Effects of Estrogen Treatment on Sexual Behavior in Male-to-Female Transsexuals: Experimental and Clinical Observation," *Archives of Sexual Behavior 14*, no. 1 (1985): 29–40.

p. 114: *Despite new concerns such as an increased prevalence...* A. Kaida et al., "The Relationship between HAART Use and Sexual Activity among HIV-Positive Women of Reproductive Age in Brazil, South Africa, and Uganda," *AIDS Care 20*, no. 1 (2008): 21–25; N. Crepaz, T. A. Hart, and G. Marks, "Highly Active Antiretroviral Therapy and Sexual Risk Behavior: A Meta Analytic Review," *JAMA 292*, no. 2 (2004): 224–36.

p. 114: *There is, in fact, some evidence...* H. Lamba et al., "Antiretroviral Therapy Is Associated with Sexual Dysfunction and with Increased Serum Oestradiol Levels in Men," *International Journal of STD and AIDS 15*, no. 4 (2004): 234–37.

p. 118: *While there is no doubt that these substances...* K. Palmer, H. Inskip, and D. Coggon, "Dementia and Occupational Exposure to Organic Solvents," *Occupational and Environmental Medicine 55*, no. 10 (1998): 712–15; F. D. Dick, "Solvent Neurotoxicity," *Occupational and Environmental Medicine 63*, no. 3 (2006): 221–26.

p. 118: *Additionally, other types of pre-dementias are thought to be...* A. Nath et al., "Acceleration of HIV Dementia with Methamphetamine and Cocaine," *Journal of NeuroVirology 7*, no. 1 (2001): 66–71.

p. 119: *The result of this practice is similar...* F. D. Dick, "Solvent Neurotoxicity," *Occupational and Environmental Medicine 63*, no. 3 (2006): 221–26.

p. 120: *And while there is some data...* S. Gupta and J. Warner, "Alcohol-Related Dementia: A 21st-Century Silent Epidemic?" *The British Journal of Psychiatry 193*, no. 5 (2008): 351–53.

p. 120: *...it has been estimated in one study...* W. M. van der Flier and P. Scheltens, "Epidemiology and Risk Factors of Dementia," *Journal of Neurology, Neurosurgery, and Psychiatry 76*, Supp. 5 (2005): v2–v7.

p. 122: *It is also important to note...* I. Aeberli et al., "Low to Moderate Sugar-Sweetened Beverage Consumption Impairs Glucose and Lipid Metabolism and Promotes Inflammation in Healthy Young Men: A Randomized Controlled Trial," *American Journal of Clinical Nutrition 94*, no. 2 (2011): 479–85.

p. 123: *However, new evidence suggests that even Alzheimer's...* K. Talbot et al.," Demonstrated Brain Insulin Resistance in Alzheimer's Disease Patients Is Associated with IGF-1 Resistance, IRS-1 Dysregulation, and Cognitive Decline," *Journal of Clinical Investigation 122*, no. 4 (2012): 1316–18.

## CHAPTER NINE

p. 136: *In 2012, only 12.8 percent of Americans in hospice care...* National Hospice and Palliative Care Organization, NHPCO's *Facts and Figures, Hospice Care in America*, 2013 Edition, www.nhpco.org/sites/default/files/public/Statistics_Research/2013_Facts_Figures

.pdf; Paula Span, "End-of-Life Care for Patients with Advanced Dementia," *The New Old Age (blog)*, New York Times, November 2, 2010, http://newoldage.blogs.nytimes.com/2010/11/02/end-of-life-care-for-patients-with-advanced-dementia/?_r=0.

p. 143: *There is some data to suggest that some antihistamine…* B. Aukst-Margetić and B. Margetić, "An Open-Label Series Using Loratadine for the Treatment of Sexual Dysfunction Associated with Selective Serotonin Reuptake Inhibitors," *Progress in Neuropsychopharmacology and Biological Psychiatry 29*, no. 5 (2005): 754–56.

p. 147: *While the risk of death…* L. S. Schneider, K. S. Dagerman, and P. Insel, "Risk of Death with Atypical Antipsychotic Drug Treatment for Dementia—Meta-Analysis of Randomized Placebo-Controlled Trials," *JAMA 294*, no. 15 (2005): 1934–43.

p. 147: *Other studies and even large recent…* Heii Arai et al., "Risk of Mortality Associated with Antipsychotics in Patients with Dementia: A Prospective Cohort Study," Poster presentation, 2013 Annual Meeting of the American Association for Geriatric Psychiatry; March 14–17, 2013; Los Angeles, California.

p. 149: *A review of the literature supports…* S. D. Moffat, "Effects of testosterone on cognitive and brain aging in elderly men," *Annals of the New York Academy of Science 1055*, no. 1 (2006): 80–92.

p. 149: *… as do other studies…* J. Holland, S. Bandelow, and E. Hogervorst, "Testosterone Levels and Cognition in Elderly Men: A Review," *Maturitas 69*, no. 4 (2011): 322–37.

p. 149: *While one review suggests…* G. K. Gouras et al., "Testosterone Reduces Neuronal Secretion of Alzheimer's β-Amyloid Peptides," *Proceedings of the National Academy of Sciences 97*, no. 3 (2000): 1202–05.

p. 149: *A study of testosterone replacement …* P. H. Lu et al., "Effects of Testosterone on Cognition and Mood in Male Patients with Mild Alzheimer's Disease and Healthy Elderly Men," *Archives of Neurology 63*, no. 2 (2006): 177–85.

p. 149: *Even women have been the subjects…* E. Hogervorst, "Prevention of Dementia with Sex Hormones: A Focus on Testosterone and Cognition in Women," *Minerva Medica 103*, no. 5 (2012): 353–59.

p. 149: *While mention is made in one study…* Sanjay Asthana et al., "High-Dose Estradiol Improves Cognition for Women with

Alzheimer's Disease: Results of a Randomized Study," Neurology 57, no. 4 (2001): 605–12; S.C. Waring et al., "Postmenopausal estrogen replacement therapy and risk of AD: a population-based study," Neurology 52, no. 5 (1999): 965–70.

p. 150: *...a more recent article provides an interesting review...* Cynthia Gorney, "The Estrogen Dilemma," *The New York Times Magazine* (April 14, 2010).

p. 150: *There are articles that suggest...* Ray Norbury et al., "The Neuroprotective Effects of Estrogen on the Aging Brain," *Experimental Gerontology 38* (2003): 109–17.

p. 150: *Also, reviews suggest that estrogen...* Larry W. Baum, "Sex, Hormones, and Alzheimer's Disease," *The Journals of Gerontology, Series A: Biological Sciences and Medical Sciences 60,* no. 6 (2005): 736–43.

## CHAPTER TEN

p. 153: *A recent newspaper article...* Pam Belluck, "Dementia's Signs May Come Early," *The New York Times,* National Section (July 18, 2013).

p. 154: *This figure includes everything...* www.examiner.com/skin-care-in-nashville/skin-care-industry-booming-with-baby-boomers-from-80-billion-to-114-billion

p. 155: *My estimate is that one third of the deaths...* Melonie Heron, "Deaths: Leading Causes for 2007," *National Vital Statistics Reports 59,* no. 8 (2011). www.cdc.gov/nchs/data/nvsr/nvsr59/nvsr59_08.pdf

p. 156: *The website of the American Psychological Association...* www.apa.org/pi/aging/resources/guides/sexuality.aspx

p. 161: *Some work is being done exploring...* A. J. Astell et al., "Using a Touch Screen Computer to Support Relationships between People with Dementia and Caregivers," *Interacting with Computers 22,* no. 4 (2010): 267–75.

p. 162: *John Portmann, a professor of religious studies...* John Portmann, *The Ethics of Sex and Alzheimer's* (New York: Routledge, 2013).

# Acknowledgments

Many people were involved in the creation of this book. I'd like to particularly thank Susan Suffes for her editing sensibility and skill; Regina Ryan, my literary agent, for helping me to get this project off the ground; and the monthly roundtable group at Auburn MultiCare Medical Center, where this book was born.

# Index

# About the Author

Dr. Douglas Wornell, a geriatric neuropsychiatrist with a large practice in the Seattle-Tacoma area of Washington State, has participated in the treatment of over 20,000 dementia patients in the past 10 years and has given over 200 presentations on geriatric psychiatry. He is the medical director of the Behavioral Wellness Center at Auburn MultiCare Medical Center and the director of Wornell Psychiatry and Associates, a geriatric and neuropsychiatric consultative service through which he provides advice to 23 long-term care facilities.

Brookdale Senior Living, which is one of the largest assisted-living dementia care organizations in the country, named him the Caregiver of the Year in 2010. At the 2011 Washington State Alzheimer's caregiver's conference, sponsored by the University of Washington, he was cospeaker with CBS correspondent Barry Petersen.

Dr. Wornell received his bachelor's degree in chemistry at the University of Puget Sound and his medical degree at the University of Miami. In New York City, he did his internship in general surgery at the Albert Einstein College of Medicine, and his residency in psychiatry at St. Luke's-Roosevelt Hospital Center. He became the director of psychiatric emergency services for St. Luke's–Roosevelt Hospital Center and assistant clinical professor of psychiatry at Columbia University College of Physicians and Surgeons.

Dr. Wornell is the author of the book *Wandering Explorers: Practical Dementia for Families and Caregivers*. He lives with his family in Tacoma, Washington.

www.DougWornell.com